Atlas of Strobolaryngoscopy

Wen Xu

Atlas of Strobolaryngoscopy

Laryngeal Disorders

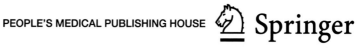

PMPH

PEOPLE'S MEDICAL PUBLISHING HOUSE

Springer

Wen Xu
Department of Otorhinolaryngology-Head and Neck Surgery
Beijing Tongren Hospital, Capital Medical University
Beijing
China

ISBN 978-981-13-6410-5   ISBN 978-981-13-6408-2   (eBook)
https://doi.org/10.1007/978-981-13-6408-2

This Springer imprint is published by the registered company Springer Nature Singapore Pte Ltd. The registered company address is: 152 Beach Road, #21-01/04 Gateway East, Singapore 189721, Singapore

Preface

With the acceleration of modern social process, the increase of various stimulation factors, and the quickening of people's living rhythm, the incidence of pharyngolaryngeal diseases has increased significantly. The physiological functions of larynx and pharynx are complex and important, including phonation, respiration, swallowing, and immune defense. Due to the deep location of the pharynx and larynx, endoscopic observation is often required. Endoscopic examination is the basis for making diagnosis of pharyngolaryngeal diseases, including indirect laryngoscopy, flexible laryngoscopy, electrolaryngoscopy, strobolaryngoscopy, narrow-band imaging endoscopy, and direct laryngoscopy. It is known to all that vocal fold vibration is the basis of phonation. However, regular laryngoscopy is unable to inspect the high-speed vibration of vocal fold during phonation. Besides the observation of laryngeal and hypopharyngeal structure and lesions, the greatest advantage of strobolaryngoscopy is the ability to acquire multiple information of vocal fold vibratory features through inspecting the high-speed vocal fold vibration in "slow motion," which makes strobolaryngoscopy able to evaluate the anatomical and functional characteristics. Strobolaryngoscopy provides new diagnostic and research methods for normal and abnormal voice function assessment. Strobolaryngoscopy also plays an important role in clinical voice function assessment and diagnosis of voice disorders. Strobolaryngoscopy has been widely used in clinical diagnosis of pharyngolaryngeal diseases and has become an essential examination for the assessment of voice disorders. However, due to the lack of specialized knowledge and operational skills, doctors in many countries have not yet fully mastered the interpretation of strobolaryngoscopic results. It is necessary to deepen the understanding of strobolaryngoscopy in many hospitals.

This book is dedicated to the deep interpretation of strobolaryngoscopy. The book is presented into two parts: the first part is the overview of the strobolaryngoscopy, and the second part focuses on the strobolaryngoscopic signs of common pharyngolaryngeal diseases. The former contains the principles, equipments, parameter setup, operational procedures and tips, observation parameters, and precautions of strobolaryngoscopy. The latter covers strobolaryngoscopic signs and diagnostic key points of over 30 kinds of those common pharyngolaryngeal diseases, together with the corresponding strobolaryngoscopic videos.

In this book, there are over 300 high-resolution strobolaryngoscopic images of various kinds of pharyngolaryngeal disease. They are all from carefully selected representative cases. The corresponding captions are concise and comprehensive, which cover the medical history and detailed description of strobolaryngoscopic signs. Another feature of this book is that there are 18 strobolaryngoscopic videos included in the book. The readers can watch the dynamic strobolaryngoscopic videos simply by scanning the QR code. This allows readers to observe the vibratory characteristics of vocal folds and grasp the diagnostic key points of strobolaryngoscopy.

I wish this book would provide a refined and practicable reference about strobolaryngoscopy and interpretation of pharyngolaryngeal diseases for young doctors, primary care physicians, and graduate students of otolaryngology.

Beijing, China   Wen Xu
March, 2017

Acknowledgment

I am very grateful to my colleagues at the Department of Otorhinolaryngology-Head and Neck Surgery, Beijing Tongren Hospital, Capital Medical University, China: Liyu Cheng, MD, Rong Hu, MD, Jieyu Lu, MD, Haizhou Wang, MD, Jing Yang, MD, Qijuan Zou, MD; and also Yun Li, MD, from the Second Affiliated Hospital, Zhejiang University School of Medicine, China. They have provided tremendous support in various domains in the preparation of this book. This book would not have been completed without their support and hard work. It is truly my honor to work with this competent and supportive team.

I extend my thanks to Dr. Estella Ma (Associate Professor, Co-Director of Voice Research Laboratory, The University of Hong Kong, China) and Professor Edwin Yiu (Professor, Co-Director of Voice Research Laboratory, The University of Hong Kong, China) who have provided expert support with the content of this book.

Special thanks are due to all patients for their generous contributions of the strobolaryngoscopic images and videos. All the photos and video clips have obtained permissions for publication from the patients or their parent/guardian (for patients under the age of 16).

Last but not least, I would like to express my deepest gratitude to my mentor Professor Demin Han (Professor, Academician of the Chinese Academy of Engineering, Director of ENT Center, Beijing Tongren Hospital, Capital Medical University, China) for his wisdoms, advice, and enlightenment throughout the years.

Contents

Part I Laryngopharyngeal Endoscopy: An Overview

1 Laryngopharyngeal Endoscopy   3
   1.1   Indirect Laryngoscopy   3
   1.2   Flexible Laryngoscopy and Electrolaryngoscopy   3
   1.3   Narrow Band Imaging Endoscopy   4
   1.4   Strobolaryngoscopy   4

2 Strobolaryngoscopy   7
   2.1   Theoretical Background and Procedures   7
       2.1.1   Theoretical Background   7
       2.1.2   Procedures   7
       2.1.3   Stroboscopy Parameters   8
       2.1.4   Precautions   11
   2.2   Voice Assessment Profile   11
       2.2.1   Case 1 Voice Assessment Profile of Normal Larynx .   12
       2.2.2   Case 2 Voice Assessment Profile of Vocal Fold
               Polyp   13
       2.2.3   Case 3 Voice Assessment Profile of Vocal Fold
               Leukoplakia   15
       2.2.4   Case 4 Voice Assessment Profile of Vocal Fold
               Paralysis   18
   2.3   General Flow-Chart of Voice Assessment of Beijing
       Tongren Hospital   21

Part II Endoscopic Appearances of Laryngopharyngeal Disorders

3 Congenital Disorders of the Larynx   25
   3.1   Laryngomalacia   25
   3.2   Congenital Laryngeal Web   26
   3.3   Congenital Laryngeal Cyst   27
   3.4   Congenital Vocal Fold Paralysis   27

4 Inflammatory Diseases   29
   4.1   Acute Epiglottitis   29
   4.2   Acute Laryngitis   30
   4.3   Chronic Laryngitis   33
   4.4   Manifestations Systemic Disease   34

5   Specific Infectious Diseases **39**
   5.1   Syphilis of Pharynx 39
   5.2   Mycotic Infections................................. 40
   5.3   Tuberculous Laryngitits............................ 41

6   Benign Mucosal Disorders **43**
   6.1   Epiglottic and Ventricular Fold Cyst 43
   6.2   Vocal Fold Nodules 46
   6.3   Vocal Fold Polyp 47
   6.4   Reinke's Edema.................................... 51
   6.5   Vocal Fold Cyst 53

7   Miscellaneous Benign Lesions **57**
   7.1   Granuloma of the Larynx............................ 57
   7.2   Amyloidosis of the Larynx 60
   7.3   Sulcus Vocalis 62
   7.4   Lipoid Proteinosis of the Larynx 64

8   Laryngeal Trauma **67**

9   Vocal Fold Immobility **71**
   9.1   Vocal Fold Paralysis................................ 72
   9.2   Arytenoid Dislocation 74

10   Spasmodic Dysphonia................................. **77**

11   Functional Dysphonia................................. **79**

12   Laryngeal Stenosis **83**

13   Vocal Fold Scar **87**

14   Benign Tumors of the Larynx **89**
   14.1 Laryngeal Papillomatosis........................... 89
   14.2 Laryngopharyngeal Hemangioma 91
   14.3 Chondroma of the Larynx 94

15   Laryngeal Leukoplakia **97**

16   Malignant Tumors................................... **99**
   16.1 Malignant Tumors of the Larynx...................... 99
   16.2 Carcinoma of the Hypopharynx...................... 103

Further Reading **105**

Part I

Laryngopharyngeal Endoscopy:
An Overview

Laryngopharyngeal Endoscopy

1

Since the pharynx and the larynx are complex anatomic structures and carry out important physiological functions, which include articulation, breathing, swallowing and immunity responses. The structures are deep and specialized equipment is needed for inspection. Visual examination of the larynx is an important clinical investigation. Endoscopic examination of larynx includes indirect laryngoscopy, flexible fiberoptic laryngoscopy, electronic laryngoscopy, narrow band imaging (NBI) endoscopy, and strobolaryngoscopy. These instruments are useful for observing the configuration of pharyngolaryngeal anatomy and pathological conditions. The high-speed vibratory margin of the vocal folds may be further assessed using strobolaryngoscopy, high-speed photography, high-speed video laryngoscopy, videokymography, electroglottography or photoglottography.

1.1 Indirect Laryngoscopy

Indirect laryngoscopy is the basic traditional pharyngeal and laryngeal examination procedure. During the examination, a hand-held reflective mirror is placed inside the oral cavity and the back surface of the mirror is used to elevate the soft palate. The indirect laryngeal mirror provides a view of the laryngeal and hypopharyngeal structures. Indirect laryngoscopy is only considered as a screening procedure of the hypolarynx

and larynx in modern laryngoscopy. Flexible laryngoscopy, strobolaryngoscopy, or direct laryngoscopy may be used as a better examination of this area when the result of indirect laryngoscope is not satisfactory.

1.2 Flexible Laryngoscopy and Electrolaryngoscopy

Flexible laryngoscope and electrolaryngoscope are common tools used to examine patients with nasal, pharyngeal, or laryngeal disorders. Optical fiber has the advantage of being flexible with high illumination power so that it can be guided to any direction. The end of flexible laryngoscope and electrolaryngoscope can approach the tissue surface for direct observation. By using flexible laryngoscope, one can observe not only the laryngeal lesions, but also the changes of the vocal tract in relationship to articulation, swallowing, and respiration in a more natural state. This inspection is conducive to a more complex dynamic voice assessment.

During the examination, the patient could sit up or lie down supinely. Topical anesthesia spray may be applied to the nostril, the pharynx, and the larynx if needed. The flexible laryngoscope is inserted into the patient's nostril and passed transnasally under direct visual guide into the oropharynx, hypopharynx and then the larynx. Flexible laryngoscope allows visualization of

© Springer Nature Singapore Pte Ltd. and Peoples Medical Publishing House 2019
W. Xu, *Atlas of Strobolaryngoscopy*, https://doi.org/10.1007/978-981-13-6408-2_1

structures from the anterior nares to the larynx and extending to the upper trachea, which includes the root of tongue, lingual tonsils, epiglottic vallecula, epiglottis, the lateral glosso-epiglottic folds, the median glossoepiglottic folds, the aryepiglottic folds, the arytenoids cartilages, the hypopharyngeal walls, the pyriform fossa, the ventricular folds, the laryngeal ventricles, the vocal folds, anterior commissure, posterior commissure and the subglottis. The use of flexible laryngoscopic procedure does not interfere with oral articulation during phonation.

The advantages of flexible laryngoscopy include: (1) The flexible laryngoscope is soft and easy to manipulate, which is suitable for patients who have difficulty to open mouth, or being weak or in critical conditions. (2) The end of the flexible laryngoscope can approach the lesion site, which makes it especially suitable for patients who have short neck, hypertrophic tongue, or an "omega-shaped" epiglottis. (3) The flexible laryngoscope can also be connected to a video-recording system, camera system and/or computer system. If needed and properly set up, the flexible laryngoscope can also be used in conjunction with vacuum suction instrument and biopsy forceps for suction and local biopsy. The main drawbacks of flexible fibreoptic laryngoscopy include the "fish-eye" distortion of the peripheral image, linear color stripe distortion on video imagery and relatively lower resolution.

The viewing scope of electrolaryngoscope is similar to flexible fibrolaryngoscope. Electrolaryngoscope has a higher resolution than traditional flexible laryngoscope. The imaging system uses a charge coupled device (CCD) chip at the tip of the endoscope which functions as an ultra small camera. Images are transmitted after being converted into electronic signal. The laryngoscopic system could be connected to a digital image processing system that accepts the electronic signals of the imaging system for real-time processing using image enhancement of intensity, contrast, and image enlargement. These would avoid the hive image of the traditional laryngoscopy and significantly enhance the imaging resolution.

1.3 Narrow Band Imaging Endoscopy

Narrow band imaging (NBI) endoscopy has two modes: the white light mode and the NBI mode. In the white light mode, the image is similar to the electronic laryngoscopy. In the NBI mode, the broadband white light is filtered into two narrow band beams with central wavelengths of 415 nm (blue) and 540 nm (green) through grating filter, while the red light with the longest wavelength was removed. This modified light penetrates only the superficial layer of the tissue can be well absorbed by the hemoglobin and facilitate clear visualization of the structure and morphology of the mucosal microvasculature. Blue light with wavelengths of 415 nm displays the superficial capillary network, and the green light with wavelengths of 540 nm displays subepithelial vessels.

In the NBI mode, the capillary of the pharynx and larynx mucosa can be clearly visualized. The submucosal capillary appears in dark green and the arborescent vascular network appears dark brown. The arborescent vessels communicate to each other, run parallel to the epithelial layer, and further branched into the finer diagonal vessels. The diagonal vessels then branch into the terminal capillaries almost perpendicular to the epithelial layer, which is called the intraepithelial papillary capillary loop (IPCL). In the normal mucosa, IPCL is barely observed; while in the mucosal lesions, the morphology of IPCL is changed and will be observed as brownish speckles or tortuous stripes under NBI mode.

Narrow band imaging endoscopy not only clearly displays the mucosal minor lesions, increases the accuracy in distinguishing tumor from non-tumor lesions early and helps the diagnosis and follow-up of precancerous and cancerous lesions. NBI endoscopy also shows the boundary of the lesion and helps to evaluate the extent of the disease.

1.4 Strobolaryngoscopy

The vibration of the vocal folds is the basis of phonation. However, vocal fold vibration is too fast for the eyes to follow. Therefore, conventional indirect laryngoscopy, direct laryngoscopy or flexible laryngoscopy cannot observe the vibration of vocal folds under continuous light.

Strobolaryngoscopy allows observation of vocal fold vibration using pseudo slow-motion of the images and provides the visual information on the vibratory features of the vocal folds. Strobolaryngoscopy plays an important role in the clinical assessment and diagnosis of pharyngolaryngeal diseases and voice disorders nowadays.

As early as 1829, Platean invented the flash velocimeter to observe the regular, high-speed and periodic motion of objects in industry. Strobolaryngoscopy was developed by Stampferat (1833) and first used for observation of in-vitro larynx in 1852. Oertel firstly used strobolaryngoscopy to examine a patient's vocal folds in 1878. Strobolaryngoscopy is a commonly used clinical voice evaluation tool now. In the USA, the American Academy of Otolaryngology—Head and Neck Surgery found that 84% of the 273 responded general otolaryngologists performed laryngo-stroboscopic examination in routine practice (Cohen, Kim, Roy, Asche, and Courey 2012).

Strobolaryngoscopy equipped with rigid endoscope, which has greater amplification effect, is most widely used. It provides more detailed and comprehensive observation of laryngeal function compared with flexble strobolaryngoscopy. However, the latter could observe the laryngeal image under talking or singing more resembling the natural condition.

The interpretation of strobolaryngoscopy needs a professional basis of voice medicine to avoid misdiagnosis. For patients with dysphonia, further phonatory function assessments, such as subjective and objective assessment of voice quality, voice handicap index (VHI), laryngeal electromyography (LEMG), aerodynamic assessment, laryngopharyngeal reflux assessment (pH monitoring) are needed.

Strobolaryngoscopy

2.1 Theoretical Background and Procedures

2.1.1 Theoretical Background

Vocal folds vibrate approximately between 80 Hz (most males) to 300 Hz (most females) during modal phonation. It can reach as high as 1000 Hz when the voice is produced in extreme high pitch or falsetto voice. According to the law of Talbot, human eyes can only sense five image frames (video) per second, and each image is retained on the retina for 0.2 s. Hence, vocal fold vibration is too fast for the eyes to follow. Therefore, conventional laryngoscopy cannot observe the vibration of vocal folds under continuous light.

Strobolaryngoscopy is a special examination technique which uses strobe light to illuminate different points on the continuous movement track of the vocal folds. The different illuminated points combine visually together to create an optical illusion of slow motion and static status of vocal fold. The vocal folds will appear static when the frequency of the strobe light is equal to that of the vocal fold vibration. This static view is useful for observing vocal fold structures when phonating. The slow-motion effect, which is created by having the stroboscopic light desynchronized with the vocal fold vibration

frequency by approximately 2 Hz, is useful for observing the characteristics of vocal fold vibration. Unlike high-speed photography, strobolaryngoscopy does not present a "true" slow-motion image of the vocal folds.

Strobolaryngoscopy system consists of stroboscopic light, a rigid endoscope (70° or 90°) or flexible laryngoscope, a microphone, a foot switch for triggering light source and image recording, a video recording system, and a display system.

2.1.2 Procedures

Strobolaryngoscopic examination can use rigid endoscope or flexible endoscope. The former has greater amplification effect with 3–5× magnification, better optical image, higher resolution, more comprehensive observation of laryngeal configurations and functions, which makes it the most commonly used clinical voice assessment tool. If a patient has too sensitive pharyngeal reflex to tolerate the rigid endoscopy, flexible endoscopy is more suitable (Fig. 2.1).

When strobolaryngoscopic examination, the patient should sit upright in a quiet environment, with his or her shoulders forward and head elevated. Before carrying out the examination, reassure the patient to relax by explaining the procedure and what is expected from them. Misty visualization could be prevented by means of heating, airstream blowing, or smearing antifogging agent on the tip of the strobolaryngoscope.

Electronic Supplementary Material The online version of this chapter (https://doi.org/10.1007/978-981-13-6408-2_2) contains supplementary material, which is available to authorized users.

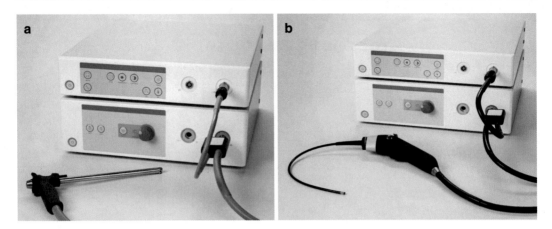

Fig. 2.1 Strobolaryngoscope. (**a**) Rigid endoscope, (**b**) Flexible endoscope

The microphone can be taped to the surface of thyroid cartilage or directly connected to the laryngoscope. The strobolaryngoscope is placed inside the patient's oral cavity, its back surface can be used to elevate the soft palate, the lens is rotated accordingly to aim at the hypopharynx and the larynx. When using the 70-degree endoscope, the lens is placed near the posterior pharyngeal wall. When using 90-degree endoscope, the lens is placed at the border between the soft palate and the hard palate, parallel to the vocal folds. The patient is asked to phonate vowel /i/ ("e-e-e-e") at his or her comfortable pitch and loudness while the laryngoscope is advancing. The examiner can initiate and control the foot pedal. This allows observation of the static phase or the slow-motion phase during the vibration of the vocal folds.

In general, most patients would not require local anesthetics during examination. It should be noted that use of local anesthetics might affect the vibratory function of the vocal folds.

2.1.3 Stroboscopy Parameters

Except for the anatomic configurations and lesions of hypopharynx, supraglottis, glottis and subglottis, stroboscopic interpretation should include the follows: fundamental frequency (F_0), amplitude of vibration, mucosal wave movements,

symmetry and periodicity of vibration, overall glottal closure, supraglottic involvement, vertical plane of the vocal folds and any other unusual findings. In normal conditions, the vocal folds on both sides are symmetric, mucosal wave is normal and vibration is in a uniform rate. The vibration pattern is affected by the vocal fold tension and the subglottal pressure. During low-pitch phonation, the vocal folds vibrate at lower rate with larger amplitude; during high-pitch phonation, the vocal folds vibrate at higher rate with smaller amplitude. Depending on the type and severity of the lesions on the vocal folds, the vibration may appear slow, with small amplitude, the mucosal waves may be weakened or disappeared and asymmetric. In patients with functional voice disorders, the anatomic structures are generally normal, and the main manifestations are abnormalities of vocal behaviors.

2.1.3.1 Fundamental Frequency(F_0) of Phonation

The fundamental frequency (F_0) is the frequency at which the vocal folds vibrate. Strobolaryngoscopy can display the values of fundamental frequency. The F_0 during the stroboscopic examination with rigid endoscope is slightly higher than that during normal phonation. Determine if the fundamental frequency is appropriate for age and gender.

Fundamental frequency can be influenced by various factors. For example, fundamental frequency is increased with increasing vocal fold tension, increased subglottal pressure, or a shortened vibrating vocal fold. Fundamental frequency is decreased with vocal fold mass increases.

2.1.3.2 Patterns of Glottal Closure

The glottal closure is the degree of the greatest closure of the vocal folds in the vibration cycle. The patterns of glottal closure during phonation can be described as: complete closure, spindle gap, hourglass gap, anterior gap, posterior gap, irregularity fissure, incomplete closure (Fig. 2.2). In normal subjects, vocal folds usually have complete closure in the closed phase. A small posterior glottis chink may be present between the vocal processes of the arytenoids in some normal subjects. Incomplete glottal closure will result in air leakage of the glottis during phonation, leading to breathiness.

Patterns of glottal closure during phonation:

(a) Complete closure: complete closure is considered normal. The vocal folds come into contact or fully adducted along the entire membranous portion during maximal closure.

(b) Spindle gap: vocal fold bowing with incomplete closure in the midmembranous portion of the vocal folds, which is often seen in sulcus vocalis, vocal fold paralysis or presbylarynges.

(c) Hourglass gap: there is contact only in the midmembranous portion of the vocal folds, which is seen when vocal nodules or vocal polyp are present.

(d) Anterior gap: there is a gap between the anterior membranous vocal folds, which is sometimes seen in the presbylarynges.

(e) Posterior gap: there is a triangular chink between the vocal processes or extension to involve portions of the membranous vocal folds. The posterior gap is seen commonly in muscle tension dysphonia, vocal fold paralysis or paresis, or is a normal variation in many females and seldom males.

(f) Irregular closure: there is an irregular line of the glottis during maximal closure. Masses of the vocal fold is the most common cause of irregular closure. Irregular closure can also be present when the vocal fold is not straight due to vocal fold scar.

(g) Incomplete closure: incomplete closure is present when vocal folds never contact along the entire length during maximal closure. Usually, the gap is large and the gap extends across the span of the glottis. The causes of incomplete closure are often caused by vocal fold paralysis and an absence of vocal fold tissue due to laryngeal trauma, cordectomy or partial laryngectomy.

2.1.3.3 Supraglottic Activity

The supraglottic structures maintain at a relatively fixed condition and do not participate the phonatory process. Supraglottic activity is used to describe excessive or hyperfunctional movement of ventricular folds or other supraglottic structures during phonation. Improper phonatory manner or pathological conditions of the larynx would affect the supraglottic structures (mainly the ventricular folds) to have compensatory antero-posterior and/or medio-lateral compression ("squeezing") during phonation. The glottis

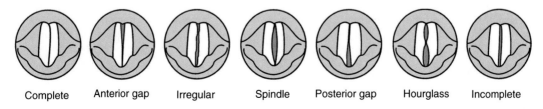

Complete   Anterior gap   Irregular   Spindle   Posterior gap   Hourglass   Incomplete

Fig. 2.2 Patterns of glottal closure during phonation

may be fully covered by the supraglottic constrictions, and the supraglottic mucosa may quiver in the severe conditions.

2.1.3.4 Amplitude of Vibration

This is the maximum excursion of the vocal folds during phonation. Observe and note the amplitude of the right and left vocal fold vibration separately (20, 40, 60, 80 and 100%). This rating is sometimes affected by asymmetrical placement of the endoscope and is hard to quantitatively evaluate precisely. Therefore, it is important to obtain a symmetrical view as much as possible. The amplitude of vibration is influenced by the vibrating portion of the vocal folds. The shortened length of the vibrating vocal folds, the stiffness of the vocal folds, the increase of vocal fold mass, the decrease of the subglottic pressure and the excessive adduction of the vocal folds result in the decrease of the amplitude of vibration.

2.1.3.5 Mucosal Wave

The body-cover theory of vocal fold oscillation has been well described by Hirano through both histological and physiological researches (1975). From the biomechanical aspect, the structure of the vocal folds mainly consists of the cover and the body, between which is the transition. The cover layer consists of the epithelium and the superficial layer of the lamina propria (Reinke's space) whereas the body layer refers to the vocalis muscle. The transition layer refers to the vocal ligament, which consists of the intermediate layer and the deeper layer of the lamina propria. Pliable cover layer of the vocal folds vibrates around the relatively fixed body layer during phonation and produces cyclical displacement. Mucosal wave is the traveling wave which crosses from the inferior of the vocal folds to the superior surface during phonation. One of the great advantages of the stroboscopy is the ability to determine the presence, absence or abnormality of the mucosal wave.

The patterns of mucosal wave can be described as:

- Normal: the mucosal wave travels regularly and successively along the full length of the membranous vocal folds from the inferior of the vocal fold to the surface while phonating under a comfortable pitch, loudness, and duration.
- Reduced: mucosa wave is reduced, and we consider the degree of reduced wave can be classified into mild, moderate, and severe.
- Absent: visible mucosal wave is absent, which is mostly seen in vocal fold scarring or malignant lesions infiltration.
- Enhanced: mucosal wave is apparently larger, which is sometimes seen in vocal folds with Reinke's edema.

To describe mucosal waves, one should also compare the relative displacement of the mucosal wave on both sides. The mucosal waves can give more information of the severity of lesions of the vocal folds. The superficial lesion of the vocal folds always affects the mucosal wave, and the deep tissue damage may cause abnormal vocal fold vibration. However, the use of high-pitched or unstable phonation often produces a vibratory pattern with no observable mucosal waves. Such conditions should be considered during evaluation of the patterns of strobolaryngoscopy.

2.1.3.6 Non-vibrating Portion

The extent of the portion of vocal folds that does not vibrate during phonation indicates the degree of infiltration of a lesion or scarring on the vocal folds.

2.1.3.7 Symmetry and Periodicity

With normal phonation, the vocal folds vibrate periodically and both sides are symmetric. Asymmetric vocal fold vibration may be caused by the differences of vocal fold position, shape, mass, muscle tension or viscoelasticity. Aperiodic cyclic vibration is one of the factors producing noise.

Besides the parameters mentioned above, the free edge contours, the muscle tensions, the vertical planes of vocal folds should also be observed during strobolaryngoscopic examination, which may also be related to voice disorders. For example, in patients of recurrent laryngeal nerve or superior laryngeal nerve injuries, the affected vocal fold may appear loose or bow-shaped. Other than the glottal gap at the horizontal plane, the level difference at the vertical plane could also damage the vocal fold vibration and aggravate the degree of incomplete glottal closure.

2.1.4   Precautions

During strobolarynscopy, the changes of vocal fold vibration under different voice pitch, loudness and range should also be observed and noted. The males have larger larynges and longer vocal folds than those of females; the increase of vocal fold mass and the thickening of the lamina propria cause lower fundamental frequency. The mucosal wave of the males usually propagates across the superior surface of the vocal fold into the ventricle whereas the mucosal wave of the females may only propagates across the upper lip of the vocal fold. For the professional art vocalists, the vibratory patterns under chest register and falsetto register should also be observed.

In brief, strobolaryngoscopic examination is a commonly used clinical voice evaluation tool and a lot of information can be obtained from the examination. There are a number of factors that might affect the visual perceptual evaluation of strobolaryngoscopic images as in other endoscopic procedures: the endoscopic procedure itself and the parameters for evaluation, the rating scales used in the evaluation, the raters' experience and training received. Therefore, the interpretation of the strobolaryngoscopy should combine with the clinical information, including medical history, the voice usage condition, the inspection results, imaging examination, etc. The final diagnosis of some pharyngolaryngeal disorders will need the wholistic information from flexble laryngoscopy, tracheo-esophagoscopy, histopathological examination or other systemic examinations (Fig. 2.3, Video 2.1).

2.2   Voice Assessment Profile

The following voice assessment profiles are all from Beijing Tongren Hospital.

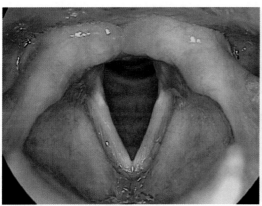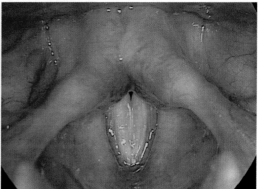

a. Inspiration   b. Phonation

Fig. 2.3 Stroboscopic view of the normal larynx. (**a**) Inspiration, (**b**) Phonation (Video 2.1)

2.2.1   Case 1   Voice Assessment Profile of Normal Larynx

Voice Center, Department of Otorhinolaryngology-Head Neck Surgery
Beijing Tongren Hospital, Capital Medical University

Voice Assessment Profile

Name: × ×   Gender: female   Age:18   Record Number:

Vocal Acoustic Analysis:

F_0(Hz): 221.54   Jitter(%): 1.48   Shimmer(%): 9.57   MPT(s): 15

Strobolaryngoscopic View:

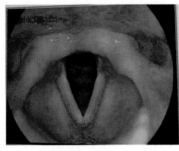

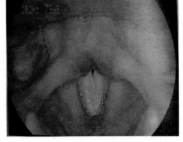

Inspiration   Phonation

Laryngeal Configuration:

Supraglottis: No abnormal supraglottic activities.

Glottis: Smooth margins on both vocal folds with symmetrical movement and normal mucosal waves.

Subglottis: No abnormalities.

Patterns of Glottal Closure:

☐ complete ☐ anterior gap ☐ irregular   ☐ spindle ☒ posterior gap ☐ hourglass ☐ incomplete

Mucosal Wave:

Left: ☒ normal ☐ mildly reduced ☐ moderately reduced ☐ severely reduced ☐ absent

Right: ☒ normal ☐ mildly reduced ☐ moderately reduced ☐ severely reduced ☐ absent

Vocal Fold Movement:

Symmetry of movement: ☒ identical   ☐ right<left   ☐ right>left

Movement: Left: ☒ normal   ☐ limited   ☐ fixed

                 Right: ☒ normal   ☐ limited   ☐ fixed

Diagnosis: *No obvious abnormality of the larynx*

Physician signature:

Date:

Strobolaryngoscopy and vocal acoustic analysis of normal larynx

2.2.2   Case 2   Voice Assessment Profile of Vocal Fold Polyp

Voice Center, Department of Otorhinolaryngology-Head Neck Surgery
Beijing Tongren Hospital, Capital Medical University

Voice Assessment Profile

Name: × ×   Gender: male   Age:20   Record Number:

Vocal Acoustic Analysis:

   F_0(Hz): 131.67   Jitter(%): 3.38   Shimmer(%): 5.84   MPT(s): 16

Strobolaryngoscopic View:

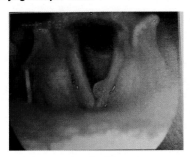   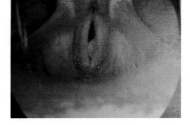

              Inspiration   Phonation

Laryngeal Configuration:

   Supraglottis: There is lymphadenosis at the root of tongue.

   Glottis: The left vocal fold has a broad-based translucent polyp on the mid-
                   membranous portion of the margin, with mildly reduced mucosal wave during
                   phonation. The contralateral vocal fold has thickened surface epithelium with
                   mildly reduced mucosal wave during phonation. Bilateral vocal folds have
                   normal movements with mucosal hyperemia in the arytenoid area.

   Subglottis: No abnormalities.

Patterns of Glottal Closure:

☐ complete ☐ anterior gap ☐ irregular   ☐ spindle ☐ posterior gap ☒ hourglass ☐ incomplete

Mucosal Wave:

   Left: ☐ normal ☒ mildly reduced ☐ moderately reduced ☐ severely reduced ☐ absent

   Right: ☐ normal ☒ mildly reduced ☐ moderately reduced ☐ severely reduced ☐ absent

Vocal Fold Movement:

   Symmetry of movement: ☒ identical   ☐ right<left   ☐ right>left

   Movement: Left: ☒ normal   ☐ limited   ☐ fixed

                  Right: ☒ normal   ☐ limited   ☐ fixed

Diagnosis: *Vocal fold polyp*

                                                     Physician signature:

                                                     Date:

Strobolaryngoscopy and vocal acoustic analysis of vocal fold polyp

VOICE HANDICAP INDEX (VHI)

Name: × ×   Record Number: Date: Score:

Instructions: These are statements that many people have used to describe their voices and the effects of their voices on their lives. Circle the response that indicates how frequently you have the same experience.

0 = Never   1 = Almost Never   2 = Sometimes   3 = Almost Always   4 = Always

Part I: Functional

F1	My voice makes it difficult for people to hear me	0 1 **2** 3 4
F2	People have difficulty understanding me in a noisy room	0 1 2 **3** 4
F3	My family has difficulty hearing me when I call them throughout the house	0 1 **2** 3 4
F4	I use the phone less often than I would like to	**0** 1 2 3 4
F5	I tend to avoid groups of people because of my voice	**0** 1 2 3 4
F6	I speak with friends, neighbors, or relatives less often because of my voice	**0** 1 2 3 4
F7	People ask me to repeat myself when speaking face-to-face	0 1 **2** 3 4
F8	My voice difficulties restrict personal and social life	**0** 1 2 3 4
F9	I feel left out of conversations because of my voice	**0** 1 2 3 4
F10	My voice problem causes me to lose income	**0** 1 2 3 4

Part II: Physical

P1	I run out of air when I talk	**0** 1 2 3 4
P2	The sound of my voice varies throughout the day	0 **1** 2 3 4
P3	People ask, "What's wrong with your voice?"	0 1 2 **3** 4
P4	My voice sounds creaky and dry	0 1 2 **3** 4
P5	I feel as though I have to strain to produce voice	0 **1** 2 3 4
P6	The clarity of my voice is unpredictable	0 1 **2** 3 4
P7	I try to change my voice to sound different	0 **1** 2 3 4
P8	I use a great deal of effort to speak	0 1 **2** 3 4
P9	My voice is worse in the evening	**0** 1 2 3 4
P10	My voice "gives out" on me in the middle of speaking	**0** 1 2 3 4

Part III: Emotional

E1	I am tense when talking to others because of my voice	0 **1** 2 3 4
E2	People seem irritated with my voice	0 1 **2** 3 4
E3	I find other people don't understand my voice problem	0 **1** 2 3 4
E4	My voice problem upsets me	0 1 2 **3** 4
E5	I am less outgoing because of my voice problem	**0** 1 2 3 4
E6	My voice makes me feel handicapped	**0** 1 2 3 4
E7	I feel annoyed when people ask me to repeat	**0** 1 2 3 4
E8	I feel embarrassed when people ask me to repeat	0 **1** 2 3 4
E9	My voice makes me feel incompetent	**0** 1 2 3 4
E10	I am ashamed of my voice problem	**0** 1 2 3 4

Voice handicap index (VHI) of the patient with vocal fold polyp

2.2.3   Case 3   Voice Assessment Profile of Vocal Fold Leukoplakia

Voice Center, Department of Otorhinolaryngology-Head Neck Surgery
Beijing Tongren Hospital, Capital Medical University

Voice Assessment Profile

Name: × ×   Gender: male   Age:70   Record Number:

Vocal Acoustic Analysis:

F_0(Hz): 107.69   Jitter(%): 2.02   Shimmer(%): 8.97   MPT(s): 8

Strobolaryngoscopic View:

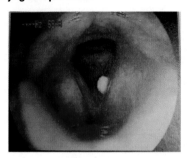
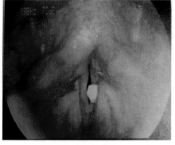

Inspiration   Phonation

Laryngeal Configuration:

Supraglottis: Left false vocal fold compression during phonation.

Glottis: A broad-based white bulging mass lies on the mid-membranous portion of the margin, which causes the local mucosal wave moderately reduced. The right vocal fold edema and ectaticvessels on the surface can be seen.
Posterior commissure hypertrophy and erythema of the arytenoid cartilages are present.

Subglottis: No abnormalities.

Patterns of Glottal Closure:

☐ complete ☐ anterior gap ☐ irregular   ☐ spindle ☐ posterior gap ☒ hourglass ☐ incomplete

Mucosal Wave:

Left: ☐ normal ☐ mildly reduced ☒ moderately reduced ☐ severely reduced ☐ absent

Right: ☐ normal ☒ mildly reduced ☐ moderately reduced ☐ severely reduced ☐ absent

Vocal Fold Movement:

Symmetry of movement: ☒ identical   ☐ right<left   ☐ right>left

Movement: Left: ☒ normal   ☐ limited   ☐ fixed

                Right: ☒ normal   ☐ limited   ☐ fixed

NBI Endoscopy: No abnormal angiogenesis is detected

Diagnosis: *1. Vocal fold leukoplakia (malignancy to be considered)*
2. Post-biopsy of vocal fold
3. Post-operation of vocal fold polypectomy

Physician signature:

Date:

Strobolaryngoscopy and vocal acoustic analysis of vocal fold leukoplakia

VOICE HANDICAP INDEX (VHI)

Name: × ×   Record Number: Date: Score:

Instructions: These are statements that many people have used to describe their voices and the effects of their voices on their lives. Circle the response that indicates how frequently you have the same experience.

0 = Never   1 = Almost Never   2 = Sometimes   3 = Almost Always   4 = Always

Part I: Functional

F1	My voice makes it difficult for people to hear me	0	1	2	**3**	4
F2	People have difficulty understanding me in a noisy room	0	1	2	3	**4**
F3	My family has difficulty hearing me when I call them throughout the house	0	1	**2**	3	4
F4	I use the phone less often than I would like to	0	1	2	**3**	4
F5	I tend to avoid groups of people because of my voice	0	**1**	2	3	4
F6	I speak with friends, neighbors, or relatives less often because of my voice	0	1	**2**	3	4
F7	People ask me to repeat myself when speaking face-to-face	0	1	2	3	**4**
F8	My voice difficulties restrict personal and social life	**0**	1	2	3	4
F9	I feel left out of conversations because of my voice	0	1	**2**	3	4
F10	My voice problem causes me to lose income	0	**1**	2	3	4

Part II: Physical

P1	I run out of air when I talk	0	**1**	2	3	4
P2	The sound of my voice varies throughout the day	0	**1**	2	3	4
P3	People ask, "What's wrong with your voice?"	0	1	**2**	3	4
P4	My voice sounds creaky and dry	0	1	2	**3**	4
P5	I feel as though I have to strain to produce voice	0	1	2	**3**	4
P6	The clarity of my voice is unpredictable	0	1	**2**	3	4
P7	I try to change my voice to sound different	0	1	**2**	3	4
P8	I use a great deal of effort to speak	0	1	**2**	3	4
P9	My voice is worse in the evening	0	1	2	**3**	4
P10	My voice "gives out" on me in the middle of speaking	0	1	2	**3**	4

Part III: Emotional

E1	I am tense when talking to others because of my voice	0	1	**2**	3	4
E2	People seem irritated with my voice	0	1	2	3	**4**
E3	I find other people don't understand my voice problem	0	1	**2**	3	4
E4	My voice problem upsets me	0	1	2	**3**	4
E5	I am less outgoing because of my voice problem	**0**	1	2	3	4
E6	My voice makes me feel handicapped	**0**	1	2	3	4
E7	I feel annoyed when people ask me to repeat	0	**1**	2	3	4
E8	I feel embarrassed when people ask me to repeat	**0**	1	2	3	4
E9	My voice makes me feel incompetent	**0**	1	2	3	4
E10	I am ashamed of my voice problem	**0**	1	2	3	4

Voice handicap index (VHI) of the patient with vocal fold leukoplakia

The Reflux Symptom Index (RSI)

Within the last month, how did the following affect you? *Circle the appropriate response.*	0 = No Problem 5 = Severe Problem					
1. Hoarseness or a problem with your voice	0	1	2	③	4	5
2. Clearing your throat	0	1	2	③	4	5
3. Excess throat mucus or postnasal drip	0	1	2	③	4	5
4. Difficulty swallowing food, liquids, or pills	⓪	1	2	3	4	5
5. Coughing after you ate or after lying down	0	1	2	③	4	5
6. Breathing difficulties or choking episodes	⓪	1	2	3	4	5
7. Troublesome or annoying cough	0	1	2	③	4	5
8. Sensations of something sticking in your throat or a lump in your throat	0	1	2	3	4	⑤
9. Heartburn, chest pain, indigestion, or stomach acid coming up	⓪	1	2	3	4	5
	TOTAL					20

Reflux symptom index (RSI) of vocal fold leukoplakia

Narrow Band Imaging (NBI) Endoscopy Profile

Name: × ×   Gender: male   Age: 70   Record Number:

NBI endoscopic view: No abnormal angiogenesis is detected.

Physician signature:

Date:

Narrow band imaging endoscopy of vocal fold leukoplakia

2.2.4   Case 4   Voice Assessment Profile of Vocal Fold Paralysis

Voice Center, Department of Otorhinolaryngology-Head Neck Surgery
Beijing Tongren Hospital, Capital Medical University

Voice Assessment Profile

Name: × ×   Gender: male   Age:71   Record Number:

Vocal Acoustic Analysis:

F_0(Hz): 142.49   Jitter(%): 14.15   Shimmer(%): 14.21   MPT(s): 6

Strobolaryngoscopic View:

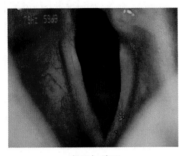
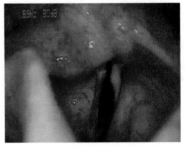

Inspiration   Phonation

Laryngeal Configuration:

Supraglottis: An omega-shaped epiglottis is seen. Apparent supraglottic compression during phonation.

Glottis: Significant bowing in the left vocal fold and is fixed at the lateral position. The movement of right vocal fold is normal.

Subglottis: No abnormalities.

Patterns of Glottal Closure:

☐ complete ☐ anterior gap ☐ irregular   ☐ spindle ☐ posterior gap ☐ hourglass ☒ incomplete

Mucosal Wave:

Left: ☐ normal   ☐ mildly reduced   ☐ moderately reduced   ☐ severely reduced   ☐ absent

Right: ☐ normal   ☐ mildly reduced   ☐ moderately reduced   ☐ severely reduced   ☐ absent

Vocal Fold Movement:

Symmetry of movement: ☐ identical   ☐ right<left   ☒ right>left

Movement: Left: ☐ normal   ☐ limited   ☒ fixed

                 Right: ☒ normal   ☐ limited   ☐ fixed

Laryngeal Electromyography: *Left recurrent laryngeal nerve paralysis*

Diagnosis: *Left vocal fold paralysis following esophageal carcinoma surgery under general anesthesia*

Physician signature:

Date:

Strobolaryngoscopy and vocal acoustic analysis of vocal fold paralysis

VOICE HANDICAP INDEX (VHI)

Name: × ×   Record Number: Date: Score:

Instructions: These are statements that many people have used to describe their voices and the effects of their voices on their lives. Circle the response that indicates how frequently you have the same experience.

0 = Never   1 = Almost Never   2 = Sometimes   3 = Almost Always   4 = Always

Part I: Functional

F1	My voice makes it difficult for people to hear me	0 1 2 **③** 4
F2	People have difficulty understanding me in a noisy room	0 1 2 **③** 4
F3	My family has difficulty hearing me when I call them throughout the house	0 1 **②** 3 4
F4	I use the phone less often than I would like to	0 1 2 **③** 4
F5	I tend to avoid groups of people because of my voice	0 1 2 **③** 4
F6	I speak with friends, neighbors, or relatives less often because of my voice	0 1 2 **③** 4
F7	People ask me to repeat myself when speaking face-to-face	0 1 2 **③** 4
F8	My voice difficulties restrict personal and social life	0 1 2 **③** 4
F9	I feel left out of conversations because of my voice	0 1 **②** 3 4
F10	My voice problem causes me to lose income	**⓪** 1 2 3 4

Part II: Physical

P1	I run out of air when I talk	0 1 2 3 **④**
P2	The sound of my voice varies throughout the day	0 1 **②** 3 4
P3	People ask, "What's wrong with your voice?"	0 1 2 **③** 4
P4	My voice sounds creaky and dry	0 1 2 3 **④**
P5	I feel as though I have to strain to produce voice	0 1 2 3 **④**
P6	The clarity of my voice is unpredictable	0 1 2 **③** 4
P7	I try to change my voice to sound different	0 1 2 3 **④**
P8	I use a great deal of effort to speak	0 1 2 **③** 4
P9	My voice is worse in the evening	0 **①** 2 3 4
P10	My voice "gives out" on me in the middle of speaking	0 1 **②** 3 4

Part III: Emotional

E1	I am tense when talking to others because of my voice	0 1 2 **③** 4
E2	People seem irritated with my voice	0 1 2 **③** 4
E3	I find other people don't understand my voice problem	0 1 **②** 3 4
E4	My voice problem upsets me	0 1 **②** 3 4
E5	I am less outgoing because of my voice problem	0 1 2 **③** 4
E6	My voice makes me feel handicapped	0 1 **②** 3 4
E7	I feel annoyed when people ask me to repeat	0 1 **②** 3 4
E8	I feel embarrassed when people ask me to repeat	0 1 **②** 3 4
E9	My voice makes me feel incompetent	0 **①** 2 3 4
E10	I am ashamed of my voice problem	0 **①** 2 3 4

Voice handicap index (VHI) of the patient with vocal fold paralysis

Voice Center, Department of Otorhinolaryngology-Head Neck Surgery

Beijing Tongren Hospital, Capital Medical University

Assessment Profile of Laryngeal electromyography- nerve evoked potential

Name: × ×   Gender: male   Age: 71   Record Number: LEMG Number:

Primary Diagnosis: Left vocal fold paralysis following esophageal carcinoma surgery under general anesthesia

Routine laryngeal electromyography (LEMG):

Laryngeal muscle	Spontaneous potential	Motor unit potential		Recruitment potential pattern	Maximum recruitment potential (μV)
		Amplitude (μV)	Duration (ms)		
TA (Right)	Normal	112	3.7	Full interference pattern	1000
TA (Left)	Nearly electrical silence	45	6.2	Mixed pattern	150
PCA (Right)	Normal	323	3.7	Full interference pattern	1000
PCA (Left)	Regenerative potential	175	5.1	Mixed pattern, synkinesis	150
CT (Right)	Normal	120	3.6	Full interference pattern	1000
CT (Left)	Normal	129	3.5	Full interference pattern	600

Nerve evoked potential:

Stimulated laryngeal nerve	Recorded laryngeal muscle	Latency of EP (ms)	Duration of EP (ms)	Amplitude of EP (mV)
Adductor branch of RLN (Right)	TA (Right)	1.7	6.2	2.4
Adductor branch of RLN (Left)	TA (Left)	Not evoked		
Abductor branch of RLN (Right)	PCA (Right)	1.7	5.3	10.5
Abductor branch of RLN (Left)	PCA (Left)	Not evoked		
External branch of SLN (Right)	CT (Right)	1.7	8.8	1.6
External branch of SLN (Left)	CT (Left)	1.7	7.5	2.7

Notes: TA: thyroarytenoid muscle. PCA: posterior cricoarytenoid muscle. CT: cricothyroid muscle.
RLN: recurrent laryngeal nerve. SLN: superior laryngeal nerve. EP: evoked potential.

Diagnosis: *Left recurrent laryngeal nerve paralysis*

Physician signature:

Date:

Laryngeal electromyography (LEMG) of vocal fold paralysis

2.3   General Flow-Chart of Voice Assessment of Beijing Tongren Hospital

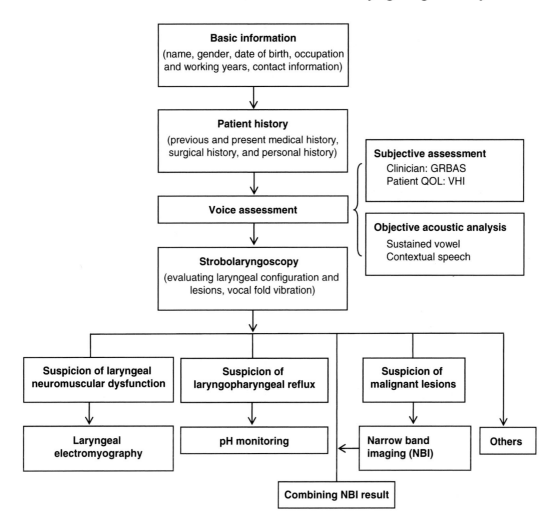

Part II

Endoscopic Appearances of Laryngopharyngeal Disorders

Congenital Disorders of the Larynx

3

Congenital laryngeal disorders include laryngomalacia, congenital subglottic stenosis, congenital vocal fold paralysis (unilateral or bilateral), congenital laryngeal cyst, congenital laryngeal web, and subglottic hemangioma. The symptoms include hoarseness with laryngeal stridor soon after birth, dyspnea or feeding difficulties. Congenital laryngeal disorders may be accompanied by dysplasia of other tissues and organs.

As it is often difficult for infants to cooperate in laryngoscopy, rigid endoscopy is difficult to implement, and flexible endoscopy is needed in most cases.

3.1 Laryngomalacia

Laryngomalacia is the most common cause of laryngeal stridor in newborns and infants. The cause of the disease may be caused by the collapse of supraglottic structures into the respiratory tract (laryngeal cavity) during inspiration, and the symptoms is aggravated by any kind of activity, e.g. emotional agitation, crying, and feeding or sleep. The prolapse of arytenoid cartilage mucosa is the most common type of laryngomalacia. The symptoms of most affected children usually are presented within the first 2 weeks after birth, and the symptoms in the majority of affected children will resolve spontaneously by the age of 2 years (Fig. 3.1).

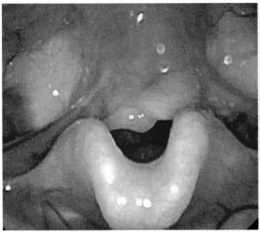 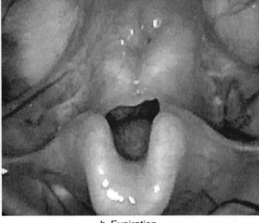

a. Inspiration   b. Expiration

Fig. 3.1 Laryngomalacia. (**a**) Inspiration, (**b**) Expiration. A 2-year-old girl had laryngeal stridor after birth. Laryngoscopy showed omega-shaped epiglottis, anteriomedial displacement of arytenoid cartilages, mucosal edema and hypertrophy of arytenoid area, which covered the glottis and collapsed into the laryngeal cavity during inhalation. No abnormality was seen in the glottis and subglottis. Vocal fold movements were normal

3.2   Congenital Laryngeal Web
   (Figs. 3.2 and 3.3)

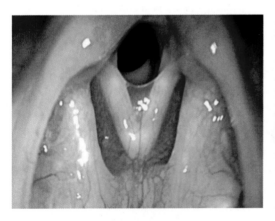 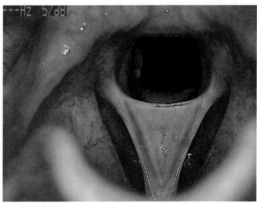

Fig. 3.2 Congenital laryngeal web. A 2-month-old boy had a history of hoarseness and weak crying after birth. Laryngoscopy showed a thin membranaceous web in glottis. The morphology and movements of bilateral vocal folds were normal

Fig. 3.3 Congenital laryngeal web. A 13-year-old boy had persistent hoarseness with whispering voice since birth. Laryngoscopy showed membranaceous web in glottis, Normal vocal fold movement but with abnormal morphology

3.3   **Congenital Laryngeal Cyst** (Figs. 3.4 and 3.5)

3.4   **Congenital Vocal Fold Paralysis** (Fig. 3.6)

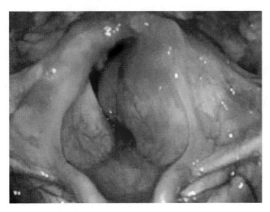

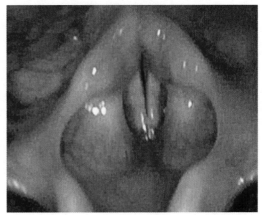

Fig. 3.4 Congenital laryngeal cyst on the left vocal fold. A 2-year-old female patient had inspiratory dyspnea with laryngeal stridor and hoarseness since birth which aggravated after exertion or sleep. Laryngoscopy showed a circular cyst-like bulge with smooth surface in the left ventricular fold and laryngeal ventricle, covering the left vocal fold. The movements of the vocal folds were normal

Fig. 3.6 Congenital bilateral vocal fold paralysis. A 2-year-old girl had inspiratory laryngeal stridor and dyspnea after birth which aggravated after exertion. Laryngoscopy showed that bilateral vocal folds were fixed at the median position

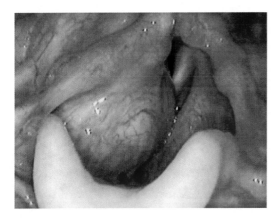

Fig. 3.5 Congenital laryngeal cyst on the right side. A 5-year-old girl had inspiratory dyspnea and hoarseness since birth. Laryngoscopy showed a circular cyst-like bulge in the right laryngeal ventricle with smooth surface, covering the right vocal fold. The movement of right vocal fold was restricted, while that of left vocal fold was normal

Inflammatory Diseases

4

Inflammatory diseases are the most common diseases in the pharynx and larynx. The development of acute inflammation usually has an acute onset and has varied degrees of hoarseness (or even aphonia), cough, sore throat, dyspnea, dysphagia, depending on the involved anatomical tissue. Very often, acute inflammation of the larynx sometimes coexists with the upper respiratory tract infection. For acute laryngitis, besides the appearance of mucosal hyperemia and edema, laryngoscopy usually reveals obvious white plaque-like inflammatory exudation which is prone to confusing with vocal fold leukoplakia. Chronic inflammation usually has a slow onset and presents with hoarseness, pharyngeal discomfort, pharyngeal foreign body sensation, recurrent throat clearing and sore throat. Hoarseness is usually intermittent and worse after vocal misuse and overuse, then progressively aggravates to persistent hoarseness.

Furthermore, the laryngoscopic examination of patients with reflux laryngopharyngitis can reveal the mucosal hyperemia, posterior commissure hypertrophy or erythema of the arytenoid cartilages. Pseudosulcus vocalis can also be seen in laryngopharyngeal reflux.

4.1 Acute Epiglottitis (Fig. 4.1)

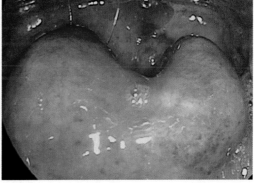

Fig. 4.1 Acute epiglottitis with dyspnea. This patient complained of sudden dyspnea for 6 h with sore throat. Laryngoscopy revealed mucosal swelling at the epiglottis and arytenoid region. The morphology and movements of the bilateral vocal folds were normal

Electronic Supplementary Material The online version of this chapter (https://doi.org/10.1007/978-981-13-6408-2_4) contains supplementary material, which is available to authorized users.

4.2   **Acute Laryngitis** (Figs. 4.2, 4.3, 4.4, 4.5, and 4.6; Video 4.1)

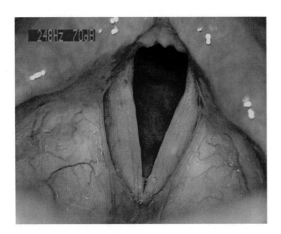

Fig. 4.2 Acute laryngitis. A 37-year-old female patient complained of persistent hoarseness for 4 days after having a cold and cough for 2 weeks. Strobolaryngoscopy revealed mucosal swelling of bilateral vocal folds and mucosa thickening at the anterior-middle edge (worse during phonation). Mucosal hypertrophy can be seen at the interarytenoid area. The mucosal waves and movements of vocal folds were nearly normal (Video 4.1)

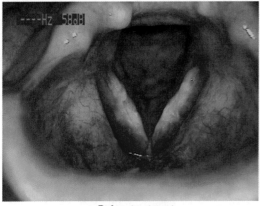
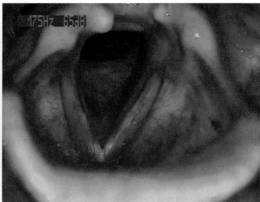

a. Before treatment   b. After conservative treatment

Fig. 4.3 Acute laryngitis. (**a**) Before treatment, (**b**) After conservative treatment. A 28-year-old male patient had a 1-month history of paroxysmal cough and progressive hoarseness with whispering voice. Strobolaryngoscopy revealed mucosal hyperemia and irregular thickened white plaque-like lesions on the surface and edge of the bilateral vocal folds, with severely reduced mucosal waves during phonation. The movements of bilateral vocal folds were normal (**a**). After conservative treatment, the white lesion disappeared, and the morphology and mucosal waves recovered to normal (**b**)

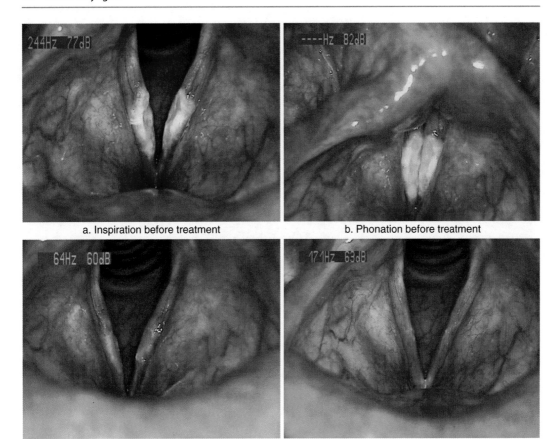

a. Inspiration before treatment   b. Phonation before treatment

c. Two weeks after conservative treatment   d. One month after conservative treatment

Fig. 4.4 Acute laryngitis with laryngopharyngeal reflux. (**a**) Inspiration before treatment, (**b**) Phonation before treatment, (**c**) Two weeks after conservative treatment, (**d**) One month after conservative treatment. A 47-year-old male patient complained of obvious hoarseness and cough for 1 month after having a cold. The patient had a smoking history for 15 years. The Reflux Symptom Index (RSI) score was 22. Strobolaryngoscopy revealed irregular thick white plaque-like lesions at the anterior-middle portion of bilateral vocal folds, with moderately reduced mucosal waves during phonation. The movements of bilateral vocal folds were normal (**a**, **b**). After conservative treatment, symptoms gradually relieved with white lesions disappeared, and the morphology and mucosal waves of the vocal folds recovered to normal (**c**, **d**)

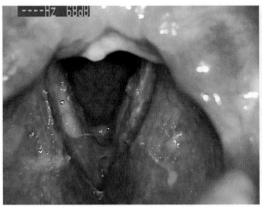

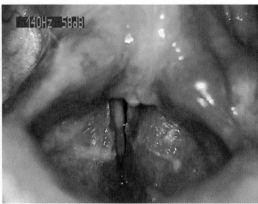

a. Inspiration   b. Phonation

Fig. 4.5 Acute laryngitis. (**a**) Inspiration, (**b**) Phonation. A 41-year-old female patient had persistent hoarseness with dry throat for 1 month. Strobolaryngoscopy revealed white thick mucus and brown dry scabs at bilateral vestibular folds, vocal folds, interarytenoid region and subglottis and mucosal hypertrophy at the interarytenoid region (**a**). There existed supraglottic compensatory compression during phonation (**b**). The movements of bilateral vocal folds were normal

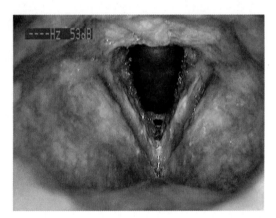

Fig. 4.6 Acute laryngitis. A 52-year-old male patient had persistent hoarseness with dry throat for 10 days after upper respiratory tract infection. Strobolaryngoscopy revealed plenty of brown dry scabs at the edges of bilateral vestibular folds and vocal folds, interarytenoid region and subglottis. Mucosal hypertrophy can be seen at the interarytenoid region, with moderately reduced mucosal waves during phonation. The movements of bilateral vocal folds were normal

4.3   **Chronic Laryngitis** (Figs. 4.7, 4.8, and 4.9)

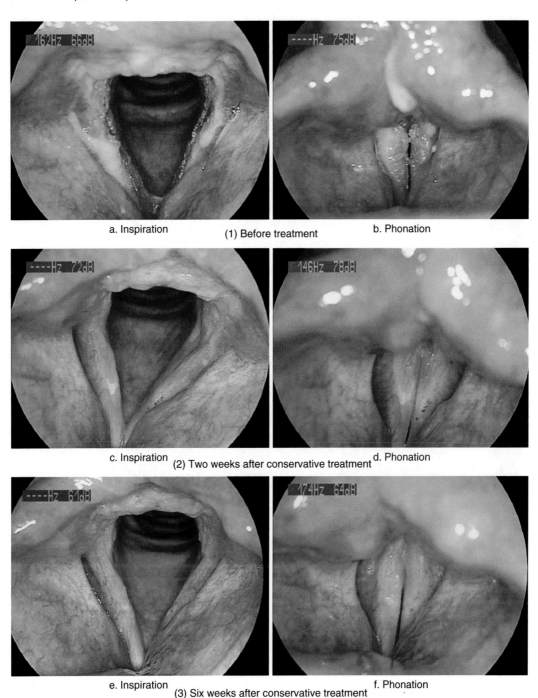

Fig. 4.7 Laryngitis sicca. (1) Before treatment: (**a**) Inspiration, (**b**) Phonation. (2) Two weeks after conservative treatment: (**c**) Inspiration, (**d**) Phonation. (3) Six weeks after conservative treatment: (**e**) Inspiration, (**f**) Phonation. A 54-year-old male patient had a 9-month history of persistent hoarseness, with intermittent dry throat for 2 years. Strobolaryngoscopy revealed white thick mucus and brown dry scabs at the edges of bilateral vestibular folds, vocal folds and interarytenoid region. Mucosal hypertrophy can be seen at the interarytenoid region, with moderately reduced mucosal waves during phonation. The movements of bilateral vocal folds were normal (**a, b**). After conservative treatment, symptoms and signs gradually relieved, and the dry scabs and thick mucus disappeared (**c–f**)

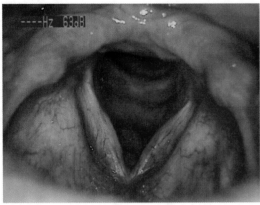

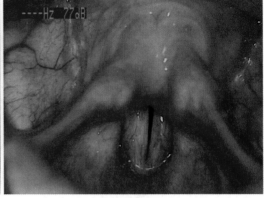

a. Inspiration   b. Phonation

Fig. 4.8 Chronic hypertrophic laryngitis. (**a**) Inspiration, (**b**) Phonation. A 28-year-old female patient complained of intermittent hoarseness for 7–8 years following vocal overuse, worsened for 1 year with vocal effort. Strobolaryngoscopy revealed mucosal hyperemia and thickening of the bilateral vocal folds, with absent mucosal waves during phonation. The glottal closure was incomplete during phonation and the movements of bilateral vocal folds were normal

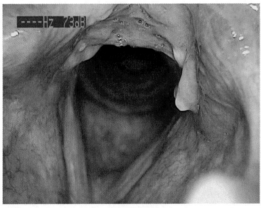

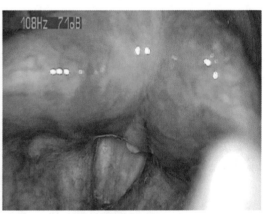

a. Inspiration   b. Phonation

Fig. 4.9 Reflux laryngitis. (**a**) Inspiration, (**b**) Phonation. A 31-years-old male patient complained of pharyngeal itching with intermittent dry irritating cough for 3 months. The RSI score was 35. The patient had reflux esophagitis for 6–7 years presented with regurgitation and heartburn. Strobolaryngoscopy revealed mild edema of bilateral vocal folds, pseudosulcus vocalis presenting at the left side, mucosal hyperemia at the arytenoid region, irregular mucosal hypertrophy at the interarytenoid region with scattered white patches on the surface. The movements of bilateral vocal folds were normal

4.4   Manifestations Systemic Disease

Systemic disease such as systemic lupus erythematosus (SLE), Behcet's disease (BD), granulomatosis with polyangitis (GPA), relapsing polychondritis (RP), etc. can also cause abnormalities of pharynx, larynx and trachea. It is necessary to differentiate them carefully because of the varied manifestations in clinic.

Behcet's disease is a chronic disorder presenting with recurrent aphthous ulcers, genital ulcers, ocular inflammation and skin lesions. Multisystemic vasculitis is defined as a major feature of the disease in pathology.

Relapsing polychondritis (RP) is an autoimmune disease, of unknown etiology, characterized by recurrent cartilage inflammation. The disease usually progresses slowly and involves multiple organs. The clinical presentation may vary from auricular and nasal malformation or polyarthritis to severe progressive multisystemic lesions. Larynx, trachea and bronchus were involved in approximately 50% of patients with RP patients. The most common symptom is inspiratory dyspnea followed by hoarseness. Laryngoscopy reveals diffuse swelling or thickening of soft tissue in glottis and/or subglottis. Glottic and subglottic stenosis can occur with the development of the disease. Meanwhile, hyperplasia of tracheobronchial mucosa, softening and collapse of the tracheobronchial cartilage and formation of fibrous tissue in trachea finally result in tracheobronchial cicatricial stenosis or even atresia (Figs. 4.10, 4.11, 4.12, and 4.13).

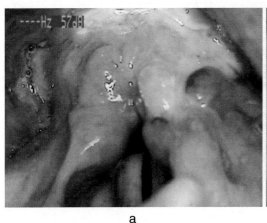
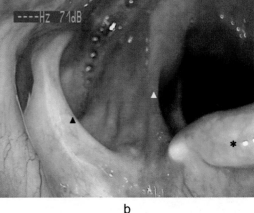

a   b

Fig. 4.10 Behcet's disease presenting laryngopharyngeal ulcer and scar. A 33-year-old male patient had recurrent aphthous and genital ulcers accompanied by a sore throat for 3 years. All the symptoms could be relieved by oral corticosteroids. Laryngoscopy revealed scars in pharygoepiglottic folds (▲) and aryepiglottic folds (△). (a) Ulcers and necrosis accompanied by proliferation of granulations in postcricoid mucosa. (b) The movements of bilateral vocal folds are normal. The region indicated by an asterisk (*) was epiglottis

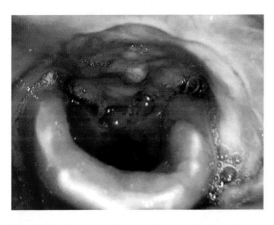

Fig. 4.11 Recurrent laryngopharyngeal ulceration. A 40-year-old male patient had recurrent sore throat for 3 years, which had been aggravating in last 1.5 months and could be relieved by oral corticosteroids. Laryngoscopy showed extensive ulcers and necrosis in both the posterior wall of hypopharynx and lateral wall of the pharynx

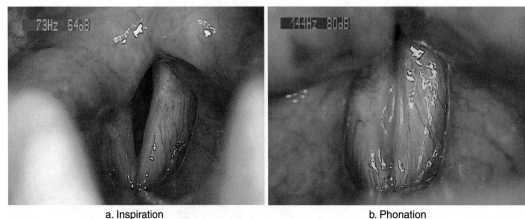

a. Inspiration   b. Phonation

(1) The glottic portion of a patient with bilateral vocal fold paralysis after the
surgery of right arytenoids cartilage excision

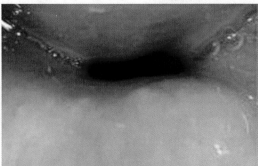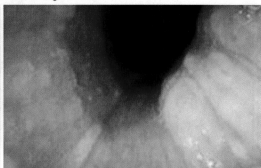

c. Collapsed wall of the upper trachea leading to a   d. Tracheal mucosa inferior to the lower end of
narrowed airway. The contour of the trachea   tracheotomy tube thickened and the lumen of
is obscured   trachea became narrow

(2) Collapsed trachea

Fig. 4.12 Relapsing polychondritis presented with bilateral vocal fold paralysis and laryngotracheal stenosis. (1) The glottic portion of a patient with bilateral vocal fold paralysis after the surgery of right arytenoids cartilage excision: (**a**) Inspiration, (**b**) Phonation. (2) Collapsed trachea: (**c**) Collapsed wall of the upper trachea leading to a narrowed airway. The contour of the trachea is obscured, (**d**) Tracheal mucosa inferior to the lower end of tracheotomy tube thickened and the lumen of trachea became narrow. A 64-year-old female patient with inspiratory dyspnea for 10 years, still couldn't plug the tracheotomy tube 4 months after excision of the right arytenoid cartilage and tracheotomy

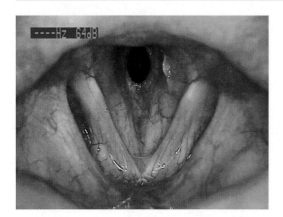

Fig. 4.13 Relapsing polychondritis presenting subglottic stenosis. A 40-year-old female patient had dyspnea accompanied with hoarseness for 7 years. Strobolaryngoscopy showed normal supraglottic and glottic portion, but stenosis can be seen at the subglottic portion. Laryngeal CT scan demonstrated a stenosis of airway and hyperplasia of cartilage and soft tissue at the level of cricoid cartilage

Specific Infectious Diseases

5

Some specific infectious diseases including tuberculosis, syphilis, mycosis and scleroma can also cause inflammatory changes in the pharynx and larynx. These should be identified with non-specific inflammation to avoid misdiagnosis.

5.1 Syphilis of Pharynx (Fig. 5.1)

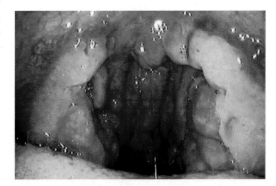

Fig. 5.1 Syphilis of the oropharynx. The patient had sore throat accompanied by foreign body sensation of the pharynx for 3 months without fever or night sweat. Laryngoscopic examination showed normal larynx, diffusely congested pharyngeal mucosa, bilateral tonsillar hypertrophy with granular surface, and extensive grey white exudation on the surface of palatoglossal arch and tonsils

Electronic Supplementary Material The online version of this chapter (https://doi.org/10.1007/978-981-13-6408-2_5) contains supplementary material, which is available to authorized users.

5.2   **Mycotic Infections** (Figs. 5.2 and 5.3)

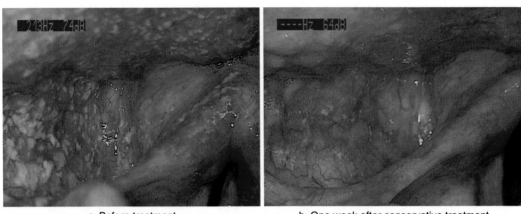

a. Before treatment   b. One week after conservative treatment

(1) The right pyriform sinus

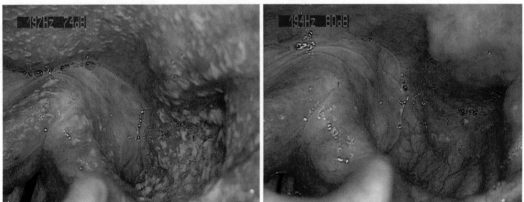

c. Before treatment   d. One week after conservative treatment

(2) The left pyriform sinus

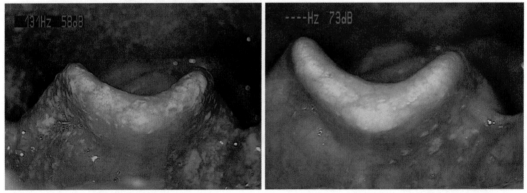

e. Before treatment   f. One week after conservative treatment

(3) Epiglottis

Fig. 5.2 Mycotic infections of the pharynx. (1) The right pyriform sinus: (**a**) Before treatment, (**b**) One week after conservative treatment. (2) The left pyriform sinus: (**c**) Before treatment, (**d**) One week after conservative treatment. (3) Epiglottis: (**e**) Before treatment, (**f**) One week after conservative treatment. Strobolaryngoscopy showed patchy materials diffused and slightly protruded from the root of tongue, the lateral and posterior wall of pharynx, the lingual surface of the epiglottis and bilateral pyriform sinuses. These lesions disappeared after conservative treatment

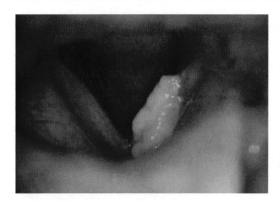

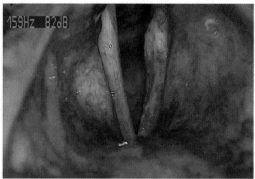

Fig. 5.3 Mycotic infections of the left vocal fold. Strobolaryngoscopy showed thick white mass on the left vocal fold. Pathological examination revealed fungal mycelia and spores

Fig. 5.4 Tuberculosis of the left vocal fold. A 50-year-old male patient complained of hoarseness for 2 months after a cold without fever or night sweats. Strobolaryngoscopy showed the mucosal wave of the left vocal fold disappeared during phonation. Irregular ulcerative depressions were seen in the anterior-middle portion and bulges in the posterior portion of the left vocal fold. The mobility of vocal folds remained normal

5.3   Tuberculous Laryngitits

Tuberculous laryngitits can involve glottic, supraglottic and subglottic portion. The glottal tuberculosis is much more common and in most cases, only unilateral vocal fold is involved. It is easy to confuse laryngeal tuberculosis with laryngeal cancer as they have similar clinical manifestations. Most patients with tuberculous laryngitits mainly complain of hoarseness. Only a small number of patients have systemic symptoms like fever, weight loss and night sweats. Laryngoscopic examination can find hyperemia, edema, ulceration, erosion, necrosis or granulomatous hyperplasia. Cicatricial stenosis can be found at advanced stage (Figs. 5.4, 5.5, 5.6, 5.7, and 5.8; Videos 5.1 and 5.2).

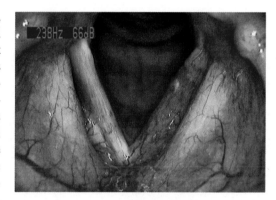

Fig. 5.5 Tuberculosis of the left vocal fold. A 52-year-old female patient complained of constant hoarseness for 2 months without fever or night sweats. Strobolaryngoscopy revealed congested left vocal fold with rough stiff mucosa. The mucosal wave disappeared, while the movements of bilateral vocal folds remained normal

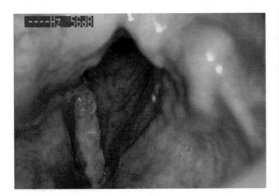

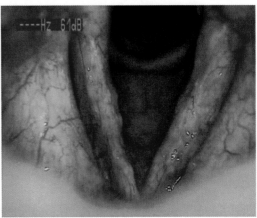

Fig. 5.6 Tuberculosis of the right vocal fold. A 49-year-old male patient complained of hoarseness for 4 months accompanying night sweats. Strobolaryngoscopy showed the mucosal wave of the right vocal fold disappeared during phonation. Ulcerative depressions were found in the anterior-middle portion with some white materials on the surface. Bulges were seen in the posterior portion. The movements of bilateral vocal folds were normal

Fig. 5.7 Tuberculosis of bilateral vocal folds. A 24-year-old female patient complained of constant hoarseness for 1 year. Strobolaryngoscopy revealed normal mobility of bilateral vocal folds. The mucosa of vocal folds looked rough and irregular. The mucosal wave disappeared during phonation

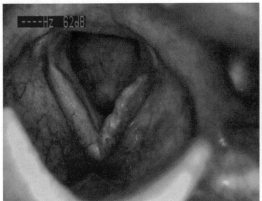

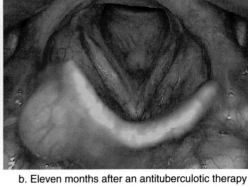

a. Before treatment

b. Eleven months after an antituberculotic therapy

Fig. 5.8 Co-existence of laryngeal and pulmonary tuberculosis. (**a**) Before treatment, (**b**) Eleven months after an antituberculotic therapy. A 48-year-old male patient had both laryngeal and pulmonary tuberculosis. Strobolaryngoscopy showed a smooth round yellowish cyst at the right lingual surface of the epiglottis, and

irregular masses in the entire left vocal fold of which the mucosal wave disappeared during phonation. The movements of vocal folds were normal (**a**) (Video 5.1). Both the morphology and the mucosal wave of the left vocal fold restored to normal after an antituberculotic therapy (**b**) (Video 5.2)

Benign Mucosal Disorders

6

Benign mucosal disorders are mainly located at the level of supraglottis and glottis. Glottic lesions, of which the most common disorders are vocal fold nodules, vocal fold polyp, vocal fold cyst and Reinke's edema. They are usually caused by vocal misuse or overuse and other causative factors including infections, allergies, smoking, or laryngopharyngeal reflux. The degree of hoarseness is related to the location, size, and duration of lesions. Abnormal use of voice can also cause vocal fold vascular lesions, including vascular ectasia, varicose veins or hematoma, leading to further worsening of dysphonia. Hoarseness in children should not be overlooked. Dysphonia in children may be due to dysplasia or vocal misuse or overuse. Vocal nodules are more common in benign mucosal disorders of children.

6.1 Epiglottic and Ventricular Fold Cyst (Figs. 6.1, 6.2, 6.3, 6.4, and 6.5)

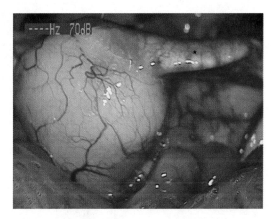

Fig. 6.1 Epiglottic cyst. A smooth round yellowish cyst at the right lingual surface of the epiglottis (*epiglottis)

Electronic Supplementary Material The online version of this chapter (https://doi.org/10.1007/978-981-13-6408-2_6) contains supplementary material, which is available to authorized users.

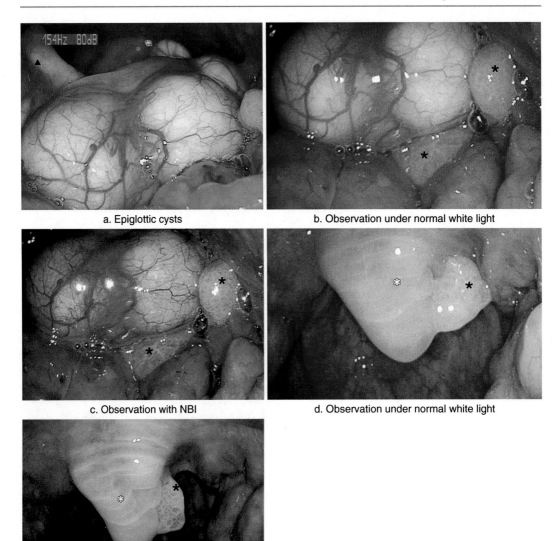

a. Epiglottic cysts

b. Observation under normal white light

c. Observation with NBI

d. Observation under normal white light

e. Observation with NBI

Fig. 6.2 Epiglottic cysts and pharyngeal papilloma. (**a**) Epiglottic cysts, (**b**) Observation under normal white light, (**c**) Observation with NBI, (**d**) Observation under normal white light, (**e**) Observation with NBI. Broad-base yellowish cysts were seen at the lingual surface of the epiglottis and left aryepiglottic fold. Pink papillomatous neoplasms were found at the left side of uvula and the root of tongue (**a, b, d**). NBI endoscopic view showed abnormal scattered, brown angiogenesis spots on the surface of papillomatous lesions (**c, e**) (▲epiglottis, white* uvula, *papilloma)

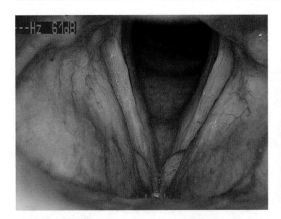

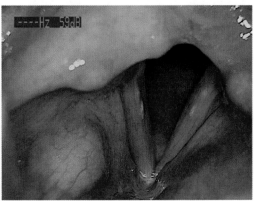

Fig. 6.3 Ventricular fold cysts. Strobolaryngoscopy showed light reddish cyst beneath the ventricular folds with smooth surface

Fig. 6.5 Ventricular fold cyst on the right side. This patient complained of pharyngeal foreign body sensation for 2 months, with a history of paroxysmal laryngospasm. Strobolaryngoscopy showed a submucosal round yellowish cyst at the right ventricular fold with smooth surface

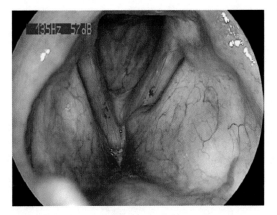

Fig. 6.4 Ventricular fold cyst. This patient had a 1-month history of persistent hoarseness. Strobolaryngoscopy showed a broad-base reddish cyst with smooth surface at the anterior portion of the left ventricular fold

6.2   Vocal Fold Nodules
(Figs. 6.6, 6.7, and 6.8)

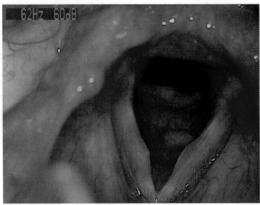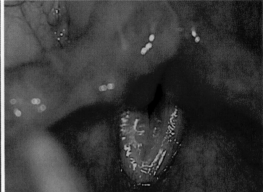

a. Inspiration   b. Phonation

Fig. 6.6 Vocal fold nodules. (**a**) Inspiration, (**b**) Phonation. A 10-year-old girl complained of intermittent hoarseness for 6–7 years after yelling, aggravating to persistent hoarseness for 2 years. Strobolaryngoscopy revealed mucosal thickening and bulging at the anterior-middle edges of bilateral vocal folds, with mildly reduced mucosal waves during phonation

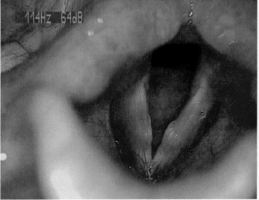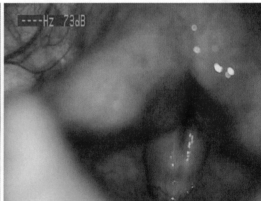

a. Inspiration   b. Phonation

Fig. 6.7 Vocal fold nodules. (**a**) Inspiration, (**b**) Phonation. A 6-year-old boy complained of persistent hoarseness for 2–3 years induced by extensive voice use. Strobolaryngoscopy revealed mucosal swelling and mucosal thickening at the anterior-middle edges of the bilateral vocal folds, with mildly reduced mucosal waves during phonation

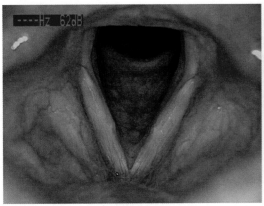

a. Inspiration b. Phonation

Fig. 6.8 Vocal fold nodules. (**a**) Inspiration, (**b**) Phonation. This 39-year-old female patient was a high school music teacher. She had a 4-year history of persistent hoarseness, worsened following extensive use of voice. Strobolaryngoscopy revealed slightly edema of bilateral vocal folds and mucosal thickening and bulging at the anterior 1/3 portion, with mildly reduced mucosal waves during phonation

6.3 **Vocal Fold Polyp** (Figs. 6.9, 6.10, 6.11, 6.12, 6.13, 6.14, 6.15, 6.16, and 6.17)

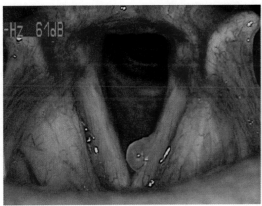

a. Inspiration b. Phonation

Fig. 6.9 Vocal fold polyp. (**a**) Inspiration, (**b**) Phonation. A 20-year-old male patient had persistent hoarseness for 10 months induced by a cold, worsened for 3 months. The patient was a talkative person. Strobolaryngoscopy revealed a broad-based polyp at the anterior-middle edge of left vocal fold, with mildly reduced mucosal wave during phonation. The mucosal thickening at the contralateral right vocal fold was present and an hourglass glottic closure configuration was seen during phonation

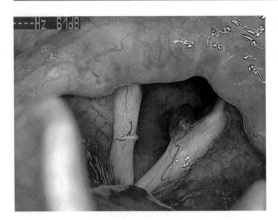

Fig. 6.10 Vocal fold polyp. A 63-year-old female patient had a history of vocal fold polypectomy 20 years ago. Strobolaryngoscopy revealed hypervascularity on the surface of the bilateral vocal folds and a white strip-like scar on the middle portion of the right vocal fold. A red polyp can be seen on the middle-posterior edge of the left side with mildly reduced mucosal wave during phonation. A prominent feeding blood vessel also can be seen coursing along the superior surface of the left vocal fold and entering the base of the polyp

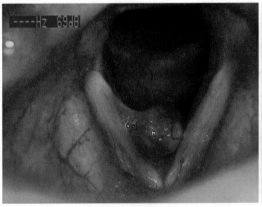

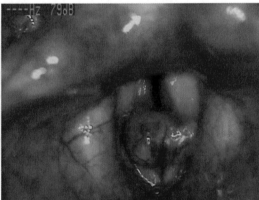

a. Inspiration   b. Phonation

Fig. 6.11 Vocal fold polyp. (**a**) Inspiration, (**b**) Phonation. A 43-year-old female patient had progressive persistent hoarseness for 2 years after extensive voice use. Strobolaryngoscopy revealed a dark red polyp at the middle edge of the right vocal fold that moved with respira-tory movement. Mucosal wave of bilateral vocal folds was not elicited during phonation. The left vocal fold was slightly edematous with mucosa thickening at the anterior-middle edge. The glottal closure was irregular during phonation

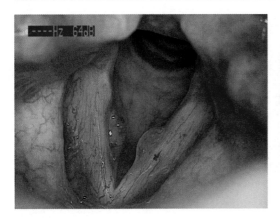

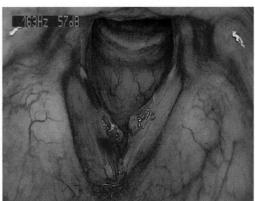

Fig. 6.12 Vocal fold polyps. Strobolaryngoscopy revealed broad-base translucent polyp along the edges of bilateral vocal folds, with submucosal hemorrhage on the right side

Fig. 6.13 Vocal fold polyps. Strobolaryngoscopy revealed broad-base translucent polyp along the edges of bilateral vocal folds, with submucosal hemorrhage

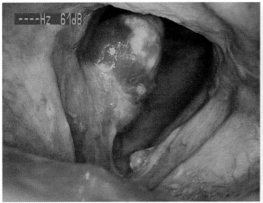

a. Inspiration

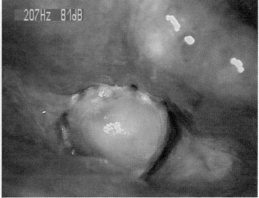

b. Phonation

Fig. 6.14 Vocal fold polyps. (**a**) Inspiration, (**b**) Phonation. A 46-year-old male patient had persistent hoarseness for 2–3 years. Strobolaryngoscopy revealed hyperemia of bilateral vocal folds. A broad-base dark red polyp can be seen at the middle-posterior edge of the right vocal fold with white plaque on the surface. On the left vocal fold, there was a dark red polyp on the anterior-middle edge with white plaque on the surface. The supraglottic portion compressed during phonation with mucosal quiver

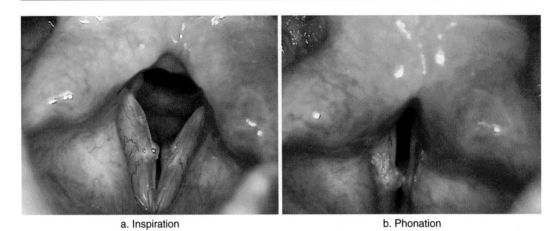

a. Inspiration   b. Phonation

Fig. 6.15 Vocal fold polyps with Reinke's edema. (**a**) Inspiration, (**b**) Phonation. A 39-year-old female patient had intermittent hoarseness for 7–8 years, worsened for 2 months. Strobolaryngoscopy revealed Reinke's edema of bilateral vocal folds with polypoid bulging at the anterior- middle portion, mucosal hypertrophy at the interarytenoid region. During phonation, the left ventricular fold com- pensatory adducted, the mucosal waves of the vocal folds quivered, and an hourglass glottic closure configuration was seen

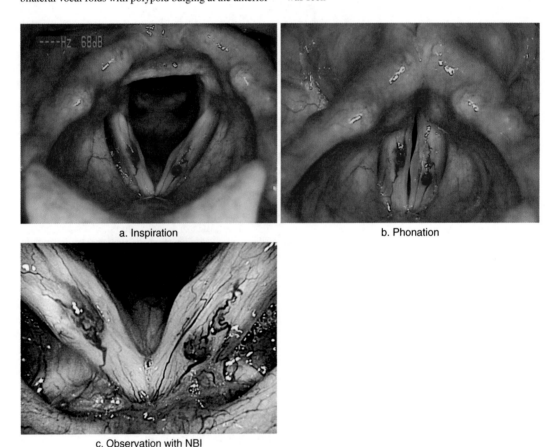

a. Inspiration   b. Phonation

c. Observation with NBI

Fig. 6.16 Vocal fold polyps with varicosities and vascular mass. (**a**) Inspiration, (**b**) Phonation, (**c**) Observation with NBI. A 38-year-old female patient had persistent hoarse- ness for 4 months, worsened for 2 months with vocal effort. The patient enjoyed shouting loudly previously. Strobolaryngoscopy revealed mucosal hypertrophy of the bilateral vocal folds, broad-base polyps bulging at the middle edge, obvious varicosities and vascular mass on the surface of both sides. The vocal fold mucosal waves were not elicited during phonation

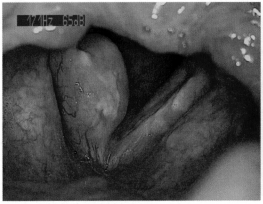

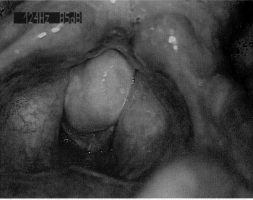

a. Inspiration   b. Phonation

Fig. 6.17 Vocal fold polyp with Reinke's edema. (**a**) Inspiration, (**b**) Phonation. A 66-year-old male patient had persistent hoarseness for 8 years. Strobolaryngoscopy revealed bilateral Reinke's edema presenting as fish- belly-like bulging during inspiration, which was worse on the right side. A broad-based polypoid bulging along the right vocal fold edge was present, moving up and down with phonation

6.4   Reinke's Edema

Reinke's edema is characterized by a chronic condition with severe submucosal mucoid and gelatinous fluid in the Reinke's space along the entire vocal folds. Reinke's Edema is closely related to smoking, laryngopharyngeal reflux, hypothyroidism, etc. The main symptom of most patients is hoarseness with low pitch. Dyspnea or episode of laryngospasm may be present in a few severe cases (Figs. 6.18, 6.19, 6.20, and 6.21; Video 6.1).

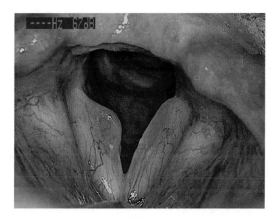

Fig. 6.18 Reinke's edema. A 44-year-old male patient had persistent hoarseness for 1 year with pharyngeal foreign body sensation. The patient had smoked for 30 years. Strobolaryngoscopy revealed bilateral Reinke's edema with broad-base, fish-belly-like bulging during deep inspiration, hypervascularity on the surface of bilateral vocal folds, and a broad-base polyp at the middle-posterior edge of the right vocal fold

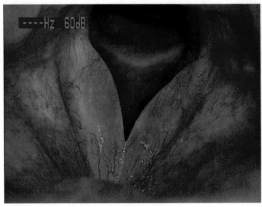

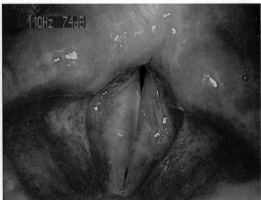

a. Inspiration   b. Phonation

Fig. 6.19 Reinke's edema. (**a**) Inspiration, (**b**) Phonation. A 53-year-old male patient had persistent hoarseness for 20 years. Strobolaryngoscopy revealed typical appearance of bilateral Reinke's edema with broad-base, fish-belly-like bulging during inspiration, obvious hypervascularity on the surface, and mild reduction of mucosal waves during phonation

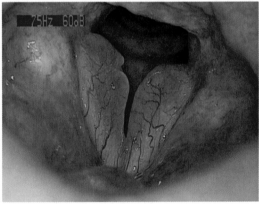

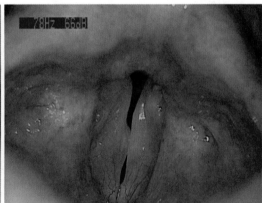

a. Inspiration   b. Phonation

Fig. 6.20 Reinke's edema. (**a**) Inspiration, (**b**) Phonation. A 53-year-old male patient had persistent hoarseness for 10 years. The patient had smoked for 30 years. Strobolaryngoscopy revealed typical appearance of bilateral Reinke's edema with broad-base, fish-belly-like bulging during inspiration, obvious hypervascularity on the surface of bilateral vocal folds, and mild reduction of mucosal waves during phonation (Video 6.1)

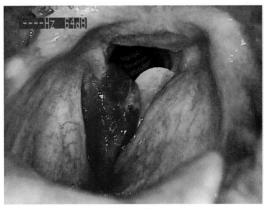 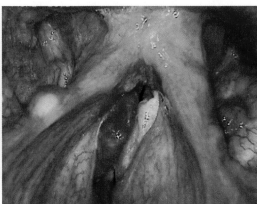

a. Inspiration b. Phonation

Fig. 6.21 Reinke's edema with vocal fold leukoplakia. (**a**) Inspiration, (**b**) Phonation. A 53-year-old-male patient had persistent hoarseness for 10 years, worsened for 4–5 years with pharyngeal foreign body sensation, felt labored breathing after strenuous activity. Strobolaryngoscopy revealed a yellowish cyst at the right aryepiglottic fold, typical appearance of bilateral Reinke's edema with broad-base fish-belly-like bulging, submucosal hemorrhage at the right vocal fold, and white plaque on the surface of the left vocal fold

6.5 Vocal Fold Cyst (Figs. 6.22, 6.23, 6.24, 6.25, 6.26, and 6.27)

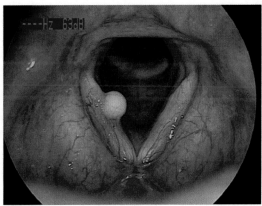 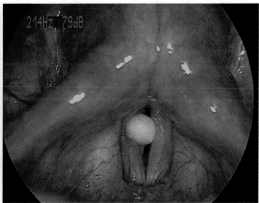

a. Inspiration b. Phonation: mucosal wave of the affected side reduced

Fig. 6.22 Vocal fold cyst. (**a**) Inspiration, (**b**) Phonation: mucosal wave of the affected side reduced. The patient had persistent hoarseness for 2 months with vocal fatigue. Strobolaryngoscopy revealed a white cyst bugling at the middle-posterior edge of the right vocal fold with moderately reduced mucosal wave during phonation. The mucosa of the contralateral vocal fold was thickened. An hourglass glottic closure configuration was seen during phonation

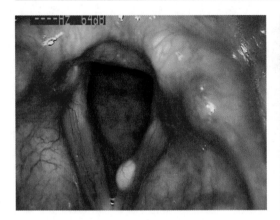

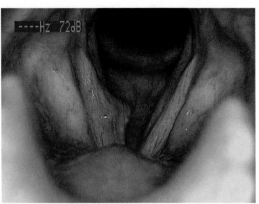

Fig. 6.23 Vocal fold cyst. Strobolaryngoscopy revealed erythema and edema of bilateral vocal folds, a white cyst bulging at the anterior-middle edge of the left vocal fold with moderately reduced mucosal wave during phonation

Fig. 6.24 Vocal fold cyst. Strobolaryngoscopy revealed a large cyst-like bulging at the anterior-middle edge of the right vocal fold with moderately reduced mucosal wave during phonation. Pseudosulcus vocalis was present on both vocal folds

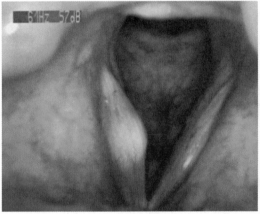

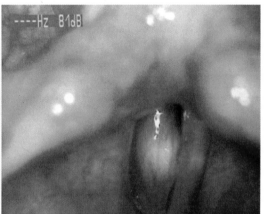

a. Inspiration   b. Phonation

Fig. 6.25 Vocal fold cyst. (**a**) Inspiration, (**b**) Phonation. Strobolaryngoscopy revealed a submucosal yellowish cyst bulging at the middle portion of the right vocal fold

with severely reduced mucosal wave during phonation. An hourglass glottic closure configuration was seen during phonation

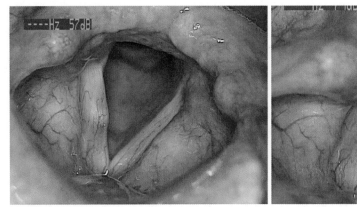

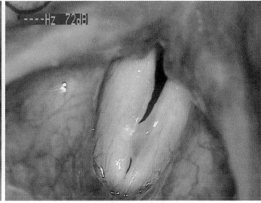

| a. Inspiration | b. Phonation |

Fig. 6.26 Vocal fold cyst. (**a**) Inspiration, (**b**) Phonation. Strobolaryngoscopy revealed a submucosal white cyst bulging at the middle portion of the right vocal fold with moderately reduced mucosal wave during phonation

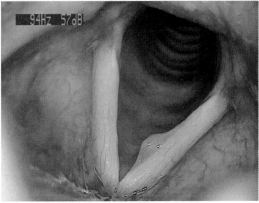

| a. Inspiration | b. Phonation |

Fig. 6.27 Vocal fold cyst. (**a**) Inspiration, (**b**) Phonation. Strobolaryngoscopy revealed a translucent cyst-like bulging at the anterior-middle edge of the left vocal fold with moderately reduced mucosal wave during phonation. The mucosa of the contralateral right vocal fold was thickened. An hourglass glottic closure configuration was seen during phonation

Miscellaneous Benign Lesions

7

This chapter describes mainly the features and strobolaryngoscopic manifestations of miscellaneous benign lesions, including laryngeal granulomas, laryngeal amyloidosis, sulcus vocalis and laryngeal lipoid proteinosis.

7.1 Granuloma of the Larynx

Granuloma of the larynx is related to multiple stimulating factors, such as iatrogenic injuries (including endotracheal intubation, surgical trauma), mechanical injuries, and laryngopharyngeal reflux. Contact granuloma of vocal fold is a benign lesion which localizes at the vocal process. Currently, laryngopharyngeal reflux is believed to be one of the major causative factors for contact granuloma (Figs. 7.1, 7.2, 7.3, 7.4, 7.5, 7.6, 7.7, and 7.8).

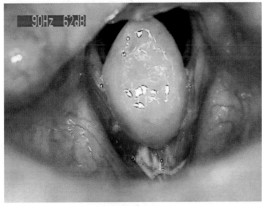
a. Inspiration

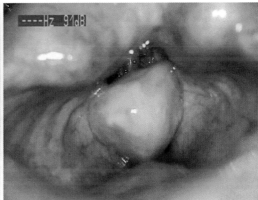
b. Phonation

Fig. 7.1 A granuloma of the right vocal fold caused by previous general anesthesia intubation. (**a**) Inspiration, (**b**) Phonation. A patient complained of hoarseness since 2 days after endotracheal intubation under general anesthesia. Strobolaryngoscopy showed hyperemia of the right vocal fold and a large yellowish granulomatous mass with smooth surface at the glottis

Electronic Supplementary Material The online version of this chapter (https://doi.org/10.1007/978-981-13-6408-2_7) contains supplementary material, which is available to authorized users.

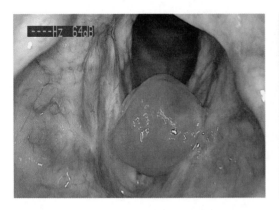

Fig. 7.2 A granuloma of the left ventricular fold caused by previous laryngeal surgery. Strobolaryngoscopy showed a reddish granulomatous mass with smooth surface at the left ventricular fold

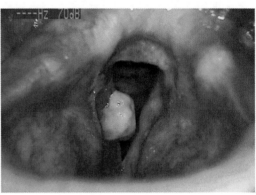

Fig. 7.4 A granuloma on the right vocal fold. Persistent hoarseness for 1 month with no cause identified. Under strobolaryngoscopic examination, the right vocal fold was hyperemic, and a broad-based granulomatous mass was observed along the middle-posterior margin. Whitish keratosis was present at the surface of the mass. The mucosal wave of the localized area was absent

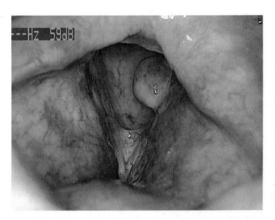

Fig. 7.3 A granuloma of the left vocal fold process caused by previous glottic carcinoma surgery. Two months after left cordectomy. Strobolaryngoscopy showed postoperative state of left vocal fold, with a reddish granulomatous mass at the vocal process

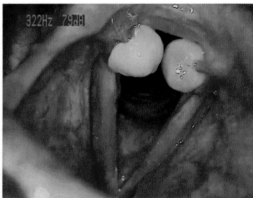

Fig. 7.5 Contact granulomas of the vocal folds. Strobolaryngoscopy showed symmetric white granulomatous masses with smooth surface at bilateral vocal processes

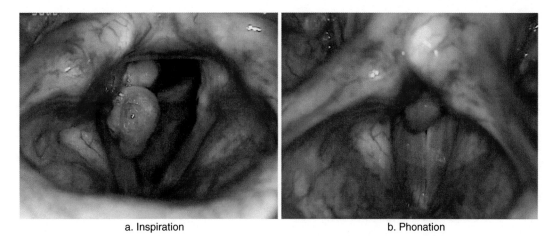

a. Inspiration   b. Phonation

Fig. 7.6 A contact granuloma of the right vocal fold. (**a**) Inspiration, (**b**) Phonation. Strobolaryngoscopy showed a smooth, bilobed, yellowish granulomatous mass at the right vocal process

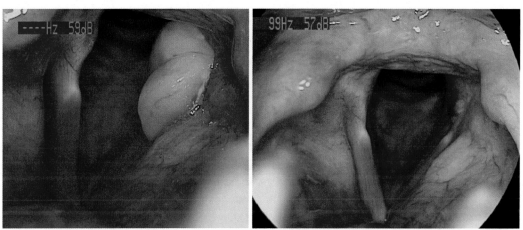

a. Before treatment   b. Five months after conservative treatment

Fig. 7.7 A contact granuloma of the left vocal fold. (**a**) Before treatment, (**b**) Five months after conservative treatment. The patient had persistent hoarseness for 3 months with no inducing factor. Strobolaryngoscopy showed a smooth, bilobed, yellowish granulomatous mass at the left vocal process (**a**). The granuloma almost detached after anti-reflux treatment for 5 months (**b**)

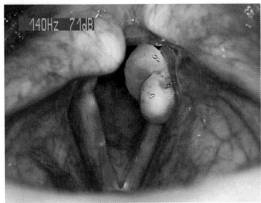
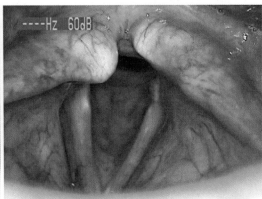

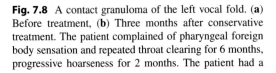

a. Before treatment   b. Three months after conservative treatment

Fig. 7.8 A contact granuloma of the left vocal fold. (**a**) Before treatment, (**b**) Three months after conservative treatment. The patient complained of pharyngeal foreign body sensation and repeated throat clearing for 6 months, progressive hoarseness for 2 months. The patient had a history of chronic gastritis for 2 years with obvious regurgitation and heartburn. Strobolaryngoscopy showed a smooth, bilobed, yellowish granulomatous mass at the left vocal process (**a**). The granuloma detached after 3 months of anti-reflux treatment (**b**)

7.2   Amyloidosis of the Larynx

Amyloidosis is a metabolic benign disorder in which soluble proteins are deposited in the excellular matrix in an abnormal insoluble amyloid fibrillar form. This insoluble protein deposits in tissues and interferes with organ function. The larynx is the most common site in the respiratory tract for amyloidosis. The laryngeal amyloidosis has a slowly progressive growth pattern, with atypical symptoms, including pharyngeal discomfort, hoarseness, dyspnea, and dysphagia. The most common location of the larynx is the supraglottis (ventricular folds and ventricles), followed by the glottis and the subglottis. The trachea and bronchus may also be involved in some patients. The typical appearance of the lesion is waxy yellowish submucosal tumor-like nodules or diffuse deposition (Figs. 7.9, 7.10, and 7.11; Video 7.1).

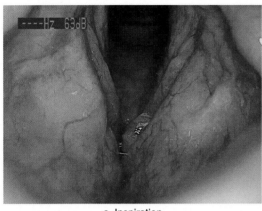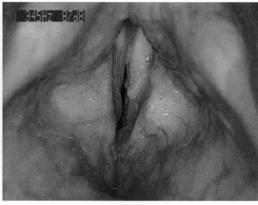

a. Inspiration   b. Phonation

Fig. 7.9 Laryngotracheal amyloidosis. (**a**) Inspiration, (**b**) Phonation. Localized irregularity at the laryngeal surface of the epiglottis was observed by strobolaryngoscopy. The mucosa of bilateral ventricular folds was hypertrophic, with irregular margins along the anterior-middle portion.

Reddish nodular amyloid deposits were present at bilateral ventricles. The movements of bilateral vocal folds were normal. Irregular yellowish infiltrates were also observed at the subglottis and the upper trachea

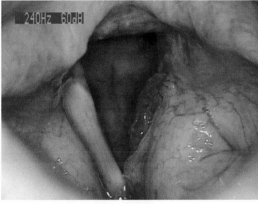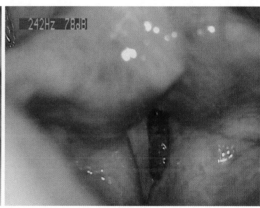

a. Inspiration   b. Phonation

Fig. 7.10 Amyloidosis involving the left supraglottis. (**a**) Inspiration, (**b**) Phonation. Strobolaryngoscopy showed the distention of left ventricular fold, with irregular stiff reddish

nodular amyloid deposits at the left ventricle. The bulging ventricular fold and ventricle covered the left vocal fold. The movements of bilateral vocal folds were normal

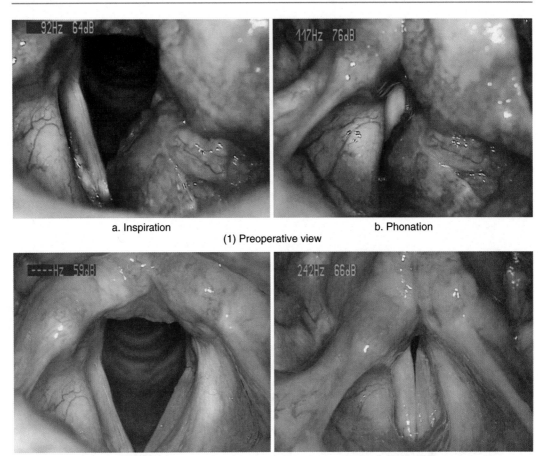

a. Inspiration   b. Phonation
(1) Preoperative view

c. Inspiration   d. Phonation
(2) One year after CO$_2$ laser microphonosurgery

Fig. 7.11 Laryngeal amyloidosis on the left side. (1) Preoperative view: (**a**) Inspiration, (**b**) Phonation. (2) One year after CO$_2$ laser microphonosurgery: (**c**) Inspiration, (**d**) Phonation. Strobolaryngoscopy showed irregular reddish amyloid deposits along the left ventricular fold, left ventricle and arytenoid region. The bulging amyloid deposits and supraglottic configuration covered the left vocal fold. The movements of bilateral vocal folds were normal (1). One year after CO$_2$ laser microphonosurgery, laryngeal configuration appeared normal (2) (Video 7.1)

7.3   Sulcus Vocalis

Sulcus vocalis refers to a condition in which a furrow occurs along the medial edge of the vocal folds. In most patients, the symptoms of sulcus vocalis include persistent hoarseness since puberty with breathiness, vocal fatigue and vocal weakness. Stroboscopic examination shows that the vocal fold sulcus form depression along the edge involving the full length or part of the vocal fold. The sulcus gives the vocal fold edge a concave appearance and results in a spindle-shaped chink with glottal incompetence during phonation. Sulcus vocalis may also accompany with supraglottic hyperfunction during phonation in an attempt to compensate for the glottic incompetence. The vocal folds are stiffer at the site of the sulcus with reduced amplitude and mucosal wave during phonation (Figs. 7.12, 7.13, and 7.14; Video 7.2).

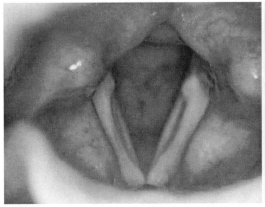

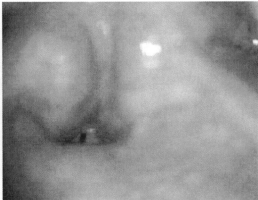

a. Inspiration   b. Phonation

Fig. 7.12 Bilateral sulcus vocalis with supraglottic hyperfunction. (**a**) Inspiration, (**b**) Phonation. Strobolaryngoscopy showed obvious sulcus depression along the edge of bilateral vocal folds, with supraglottic compression during phonation

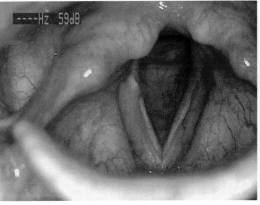

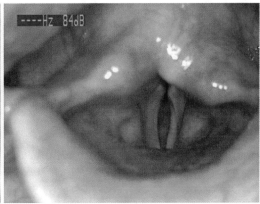

a. Inspiration   b. Phonation

Fig. 7.13 Bilateral sulcus vocalis. (**a**) Inspiration, (**b**) Phonation. A 19-year-old male patient had persistent hoarseness for 3 years. Sulcus depression was present along the edge of bilateral vocal folds under strobolaryngoscopy. The stiffness of vocal fold vibration, the reduction of the mucosal wave, the spindle-shaped gap of glottal closure and supraglottic compression were seen during phonation (Video 7.2)

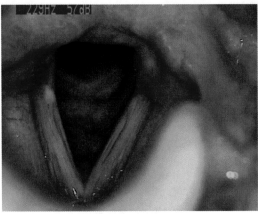

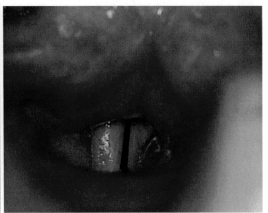

a. Inspiration   b. Phonation

Fig. 7.14 Bilateral sulcus vocalis. (**a**) Inspiration, (**b**) Phonation. A 25-year-old male patient had persistent hoarseness for 17 years. Strobolaryngoscopy showed sulcus depression along the edge of bilateral vocal folds and the left side was more severe. Supraglottic anteroposterior compression was seen during phonation

7.4   Lipoid Proteinosis of the Larynx

Lipoid proteinosis is a rare disease caused by deposition of hyaline material in the skin and mucous membranes. The laryngeal infiltration is the most typical mucous manifestation, mainly involving the mucosa of vocal fold and interarytenoid region. Hoarseness is the most common symptom and usually is the first manifestation of the disease, which mostly begins in infancy and is lifelong. Lipoid proteinosis may be accompanied by mucocutaneous changes of other sites all over the body, including oral cavity, the eyelids, the face, and the limbs (Figs. 7.15, 7.16, and 7.17).

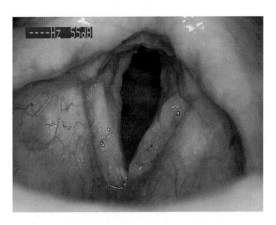

Fig. 7.15 Lipoid proteinosis of the larynx. A 30-year-old female patient had persistent hoarseness since birth. Strobolaryngoscopy showed irregularities along the full length of vocal folds and thickening of the interarytenoid region due to the deposition of the yellowish papules. The stiff vocal fold vibration and the absent mucosal wave were seen during phonation. The movements of bilateral vocal folds were normal

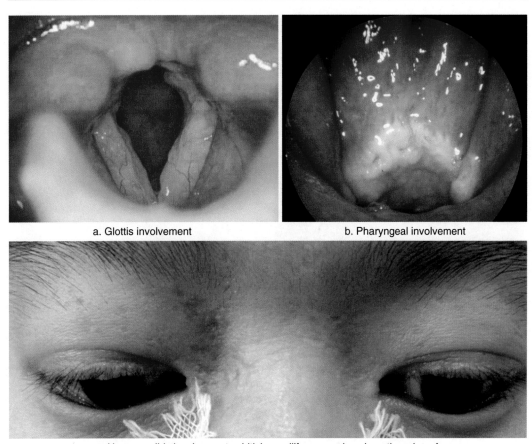

a. Glottis involvement   b. Pharyngeal involvement

c. Upper eyelids involvement: whitish moniliform papules along the edge of
upper eyelids and pocklike infiltrations with pigmentation on the face

Fig. 7.16 Lipoid proteinosis. (**a**) Glottis involvement, (**b**) Pharyngeal involvement, (**c**) Upper eyelids involvement: whitish moniliform papules along the edge of upper eyelids and pocklike infiltrations with pigmentation on the face. A 20-year-old female patient had persistent hoarseness since 3 years old. The whitish moniliform papules on the eyelids, skin thickening on the face and limbs were discovered at 10 years old. Strobolaryngoscopy showed irregularities along the edges and surfaces of vocal folds and thickening of the interarytenoid region due to the deposition of the yellowish papules. The pharyngeal mucosa showed irregular yellowish infiltrates (Reproduced with permission from [1])

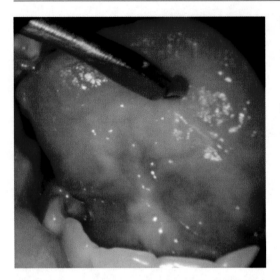

Fig. 7.17 Lipoid proteinosis, tongue involvement with thickened frenulum. The patient complained that tongue was thickened and hard to retroflex since 13–14 years old. The yellowish infiltrates were seen at the tongue and frenulum, leading to the shortening of the frenulum (Reproduced with permission from [2])

References

1. Xu W, Wang L, Zhang L, et al. Otolaryngological manifestations and genetic characteristics of lipoid proteinosis. Ann Otol Rhinol Laryngol. 2010;119(11):767–71.
2. Xu W, Wang L, Zhang L, et al. Manifestation and treatment of lipoid proteinosis in larynx. Zhonghua Er Bi Yan Hou Tou Jing Wai Ke Za Zhi. 2010;45(4):301–4.

Laryngeal Trauma

8

Various causes, such as trauma, corrosive injury, thermal injury, foreign body, and surgery can damage the laryngeal cartilages, mucosa, soft tissues and joints, resulting in hoarseness, dyspnea, and/or dysphagia. Scarred stenosis may occur in later period in some patients (Figs. 8.1, 8.2, and 8.3).

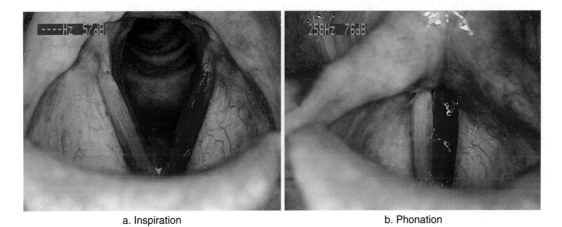

a. Inspiration   b. Phonation

Fig. 8.1 Hemorrhage of the left vocal fold. (**a**) Inspiration, (**b**) Phonation

© Springer Nature Singapore Pte Ltd. and Peoples Medical Publishing House 2019
W. Xu, *Atlas of Strobolaryngoscopy*, https://doi.org/10.1007/978-981-13-6408-2_8

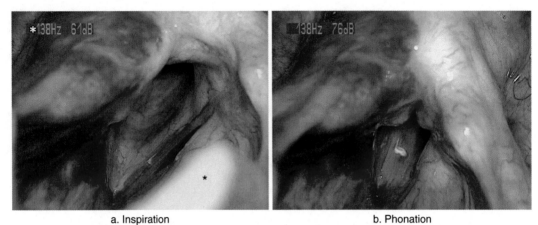

a. Inspiration   b. Phonation

(1) Submucosal hemorrhage involving the right arytenoid and ventricular fold.
The right vocal fold was fixed near the median position and the glottal
closure was complete during phonation (*epiglottis)

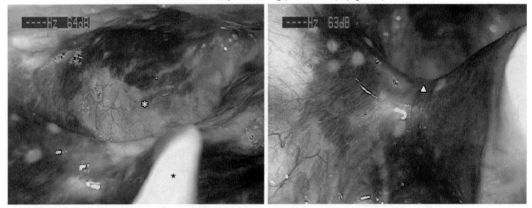

(2) Submucosal hemorrhage involving the right pharyngoepiglottic fold (Δ),
aryepiglottic fold, and pyriform fossa (*epiglottis)

Fig. 8.2 Blunt trauma of the larynx with diffuse hemorrhage on the right side and immobility of the right vocal fold. (1) Submucosal hemorrhage involving the right arytenoid and ventricular fold. The right vocal fold was fixed near the median position and the glottal closure was complete during phonation (*epiglottis): (**a**) Inspiration, (**b**) Phonation. (2) Submucosal hemorrhage involving the right pharyngoepiglottic fold (Δ), aryepiglottic fold, and pyriform fossa (white *) (*epiglottis) (**c, d**)

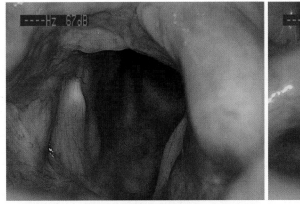

a. Inspiration

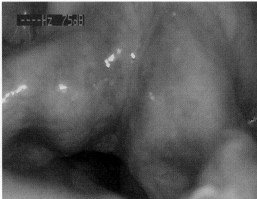

b. Phonation

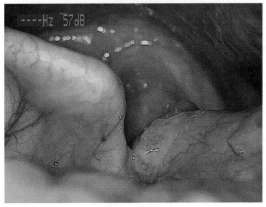

c. Supraglottic area

Fig. 8.3 Penetrating laryngeal injury with a displaced fracture of the thyroid ala. (**a**) Inspiration, (**b**) Phonation, (**c**) Supraglottic area. The patient had hoarseness with whispered sound. Strobolaryngoscopy showed partial absence of the epiglottis and scar formation on the glottis and supraglottis. The structure of the anterior glottis was abnormal presenting with absence of the front of bilateral vocal folds and anterior commissure. Anteriomedial displacement of bilateral arytenoids and supraglottic compression were seen during phonation

Vocal Fold Immobility

9

Vocal fold immobility may be the result from neuromuscular damage and/or mechanical problems, including the disorders of central nervous system, peripheral nervous system, arytenoid joint fixation, or neuromuscular junction disease. The severity of symptoms varies which mainly depends on the degree of the injury, the position of the immobile vocal fold and the compensation of laryngeal function. The manifestations of unilateral vocal fold paralysis and arytenoid dislocation are similar, including different degrees of hoarseness, breathiness, vocal fatigue, aspiration, vocal fold hypomobility or immobility and glottal insufficiency. Bilateral vocal fold paralysis includes abductory type and adductory type, and bilateral abductor vocal fold paralysis is most common and usually accompanied by severe dyspnea and laryngeal stridor, while bilateral adductor vocal fold paralysis usually causes hoarseness and aspiration.

Electronic Supplementary Material The online version of this chapter (https://doi.org/10.1007/978-981-13-6408-2_9) contains supplementary material, which is available to authorized users.

W. Xu, *Atlas of Strobolaryngoscopy*, https://doi.org/10.1007/978-981-13-6408-2_9

9.1 **Vocal Fold Paralysis** (Figs. 9.1, 9.2, 9.3, and 9.4; Videos 9.1, 9.2, and 9.3)

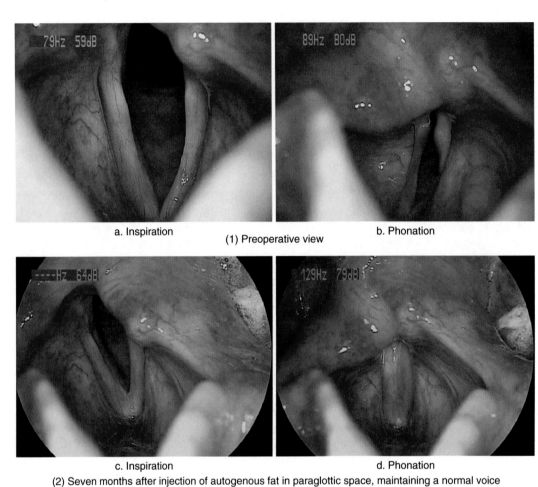

a. Inspiration

(1) Preoperative view

b. Phonation

c. Inspiration

d. Phonation

(2) Seven months after injection of autogenous fat in paraglottic space, maintaining a normal voice

Fig. 9.1 Left vocal fold paralysis following esophageal carcinoma surgery. (1) Preoperative view: (**a**) Inspiration, (**b**) Phonation. (2) Seven months after injection of autogenous fat in paraglottic space, maintaining a normal voice: (**c**) Inspiration, (**d**) Phonation. A 71-year-old male patient had hoarseness after esophageal carcinoma surgery. Strobolaryngoscopy revealed the left vocal fold with bowing fixed in the abduction position, symmetrical vertical plane of bilateral vocal folds. During phonation, a large glottic gap configuration was seen, with the supraglottic compression and mucosal flutter (1) (Video 9.1). Seven months after injection of autogenous fat in paraglottic space, the patient retrieved normal voice. Strobolaryngoscopy revealed that left vocal fold had a nearly normal shape and medialization with complete glottal closure and normal mucosal wave during phonation (2) (Video 9.2)

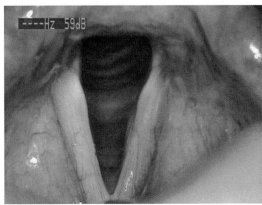 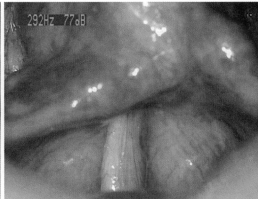

| a. Inspiration | b. Phonation: complete glottis closure and normal mucosal wave |

Fig. 9.2 Left vocal fold paralysis, 10 years after injection of autogenous fat, still maintaining a normal voice. (**a**) Inspiration, (**b**) Phonation: complete glottis closure and normal mucosal wave. Strobolaryngoscopy revealed the left vocal fold fixed in the paramedian position with normal shape, normal mucosal wave and complete glottic closure during phonation (Video 9.3)

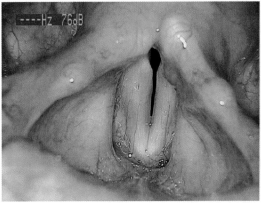 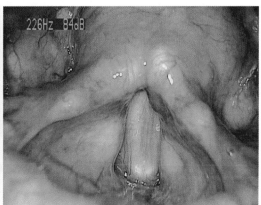

| a. Inspiration | b. Phonation |

Fig. 9.3 Bilateral abductor vocal fold paralysis with dyspnea. (**a**) Inspiration, (**b**) Phonation. The patient was initially tracheotomy-dependent with a history of total thyroidectomy due to thyroid cancer. He had a normal voice. Strobolaryngoscopy showed both vocal folds fixed in the median position and could not abduct during inspiration. During phonation, the mucosal wave of bilateral vocal folds was normal, the glottic closure was complete and bilateral ventricular folds were mildly compressed

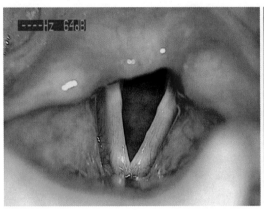

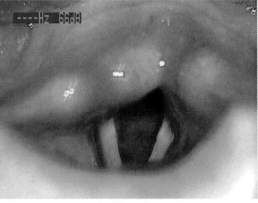

a. Inspiration   b. Phonation

Fig. 9.4 Bilateral vocal fold paralysis with dysphonia. (**a**) Inspiration, (**b**) Phonation. A 10-year-old female patient had a whispered voice after endotracheal intubation because of closed craniocerebral trauma. Strobolaryngoscopy revealed that the right vocal fold was fixed in the paramedian position while the left vocal fold was fixed in the lateral position. Incomplete glottis closure and supraglottic anteroposterior compression were seen during phonation

9.2   Arytenoid Dislocation

Arytenoid dislocation is mostly caused by endotracheal intubation under general anesthesia. However, there are also a few patients who have arytenoid dislocation due to coughing, sneezing or nasogastric tube insertion. It is hard to distinguish arytenoid dislocation from vocal fold paralysis by symptoms and laryngoscopic signs. Clinically, diagnosis is performed through a combination of medical history and physical signs, especially the history of intubation, laryngeal trauma, and rheumatoid diseases. Laryngeal electromyography should help to determine the reason of vocal fold immobility. A timely closed arytenoid reduction is the optimal choice for managing arytenoid dislocation (Figs. 9.5 and 9.6; Videos 9.4, 9.5, 9.6, and 9.7).

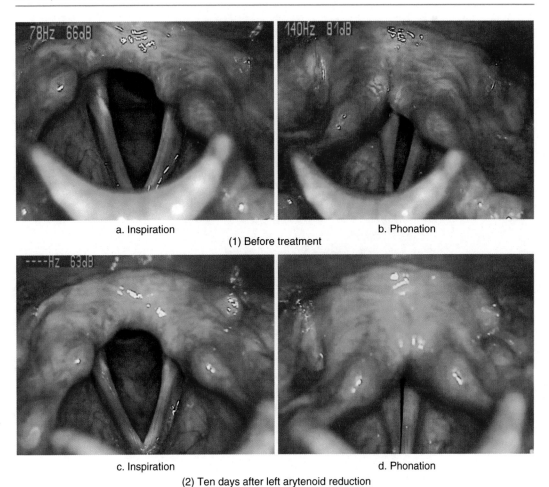

a. Inspiration   b. Phonation

(1) Before treatment

c. Inspiration   d. Phonation

(2) Ten days after left arytenoid reduction

Fig. 9.5 Arytenoid dislocation on the left side. (1) Before treatment: (**a**) Inspiration, (**b**) Phonation. (2) Ten days after left arytenoid reduction: (**c**) Inspiration, (**d**) Phonation. A 20-year-old female patient complained of hoarseness following endotracheal ntubation for gynecologic surgery. Strobolaryngoscopy showed the left vocal fold fixed in the paramedian position. During phonation, the glottic closure was incomplete with a large gap; the vertical plane of the left vocal fold was higher than the other side and the mucosal wave fluttered (1) (Video 9.4). Ten days after left arytenoid reduction, the patient returned to her normal voice. The movements, the mucosal wave, the symmetry of bilateral vocal folds and the glottic closure all recovered to normal (2) (Video 9.5)

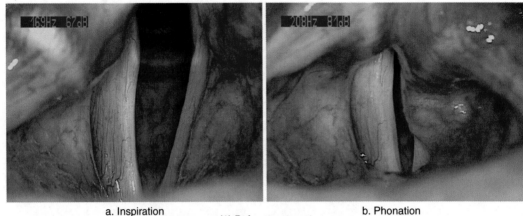

a. Inspiration   b. Phonation

(1) Before treatment

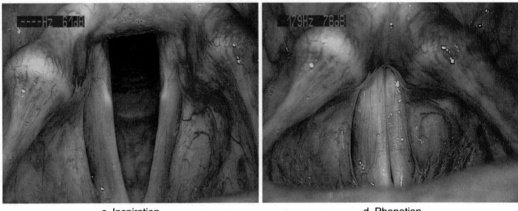

c. Inspiration   d. Phonation

(2) Two weeks after right arytenoid reduction

Fig. 9.6 Arytenoid dislocation on the right side. (1) Before treatment: (**a**) Inspiration, (**b**) Phonation. (2) Two weeks after right arytenoid reduction: (**c**) Inspiration, (**d**) Phonation. A 77-year-old male patient had hoarseness after gallbladder surgery under general anesthesia using laryngeal mask. Strobolaryngoscopy showed the right vocal fold with bowing was fixed near the median position. During phonation, the left ventricular fold adducted compensatory, the mucosal wave of the right vocal fold reduced mildly, the glottic closure was incomplete with a large gap. The vertical plane of the right vocal fold was higher than the other side (1) (Video 9.6). Two weeks after right arytenoid reduction, the patient returned to his normal voice. Strobolaryngoscopy showed that the movement, the mucosal wave, and the glottis closure all recovered to normal. The discrepancy in the vertical plane of bilateral vocal folds and the compensatory adduction of left ventricular fold improved significantly (2) (Video 9.7)

Spasmodic Dysphonia

10

Spasmodic dysphonia is mainly caused by hyperadduction (closure) of the vocal folds due to involuntary contraction or spasm of intrinsic laryngeal muscles (mainly the adductor muscle) during phonation, resulting in strained phonation and voice break. The diagnosis is based on subjective perceptual assessments and judged by clinical manifestations. Currently, intramuscular injection of botulinum toxin type A into the affected muscles is the first choice of treatment method. The author's research supports the recommendation that the spasmodic dysphonia should be diagnosed and evaluated by laryngeal electromyography. After Botox injection, the electromyographic characteristics and clinical features would also aid to determine the effects of treatment (Fig. 10.1).

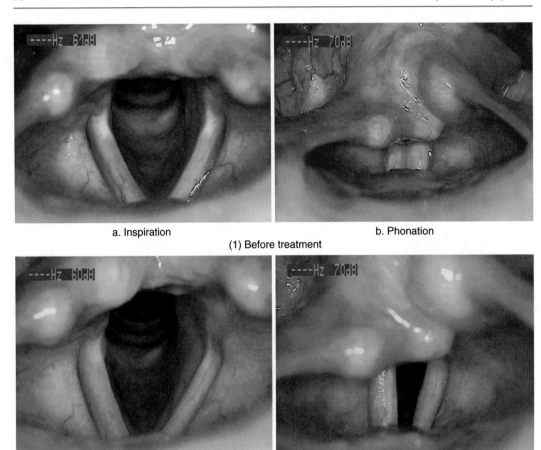

a. Inspiration   b. Phonation
(1) Before treatment

c. Inspiration   d. Phonation
(2) Two weeks after botulinum toxin injection of bilateral thyroarytenoid muscles

Fig. 10.1 Adductor spasmodic dysphonia. (1) Before treatment: (**a**) Inspiration, (**b**) Phonation. (2) Two weeks after botulinum toxin injection of bilateral thyroarytenoid muscles: (**c**) Inspiration, (**d**) Phonation. The patient had vocal break for 6 years, with strained-strangled voice and vocal effort. Strobolaryngoscopy showed obvious squeezing of bilateral arytenoid cartilages and tremor of the larynx at the end of the phonation (1). Two weeks after botulinum toxin injection of bilateral thyroarytenoid muscles, strained-strangled voice and vocal break disappeared and breathy voice appeared instead. Strobolaryngoscopy showed that vocal fold adduction was limited, leading to apparent glottic insufficiency during phonation (2)

Functional Dysphonia

11

Functional dysphonia results from abnormal phonatory modes or vocal behaviors when laryngeal structure is normal. Examples of the vocal behaviors include vocal fatigue, muscle tension dysphonia, functional aphonia, and ventricular fold phonation, leading to hoarseness and even aphonia. Functional dysphonia can be caused by a variety of factors or stimulation, following psychological factor or emotional excitement, or secondary to organic laryngeal lesions. Long-term or inadequate voice rest can also lead to secondary functional dysphonia. Voice therapy is the main treatment approach for functional dysphonia. Psychotherapy can also assist at the same time (Figs. 11.1, 11.2, and 11.3; Videos 11.1 and 11.2).

Electronic Supplementary Material The online version of this chapter (https://doi.org/10.1007/978-981-13-6408-2_11) contains supplementary material, which is available to authorized users.

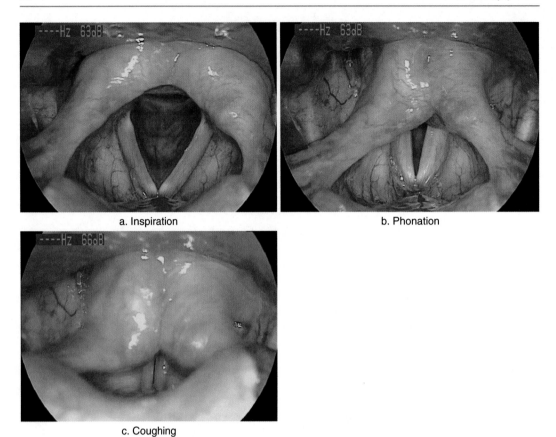

a. Inspiration   b. Phonation

c. Coughing

Fig. 11.1 Functional aphonia. (**a**) Inspiration, (**b**) Phonation, (**c**) Coughing. A 52-year-old female patient had persistent hoarseness for 3 months with a history of absolute voice rest for 2 months. The patient presented with whispered voice on attempted phonation, but normal cough voice. Strobolaryngoscopy showed normal morphology of vocal folds, with incomplete glottal closure (large glottic gap) during phonation while complete glottal closure during cough

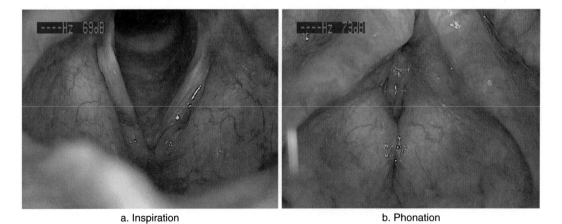

a. Inspiration   b. Phonation

Fig. 11.2 Functional aphonia. (**a**) Inspiration, (**b**) Phonation. An 11-year-old boy had persistent hoarseness after vocal overuse for 20 days and voice rest for 7 days. Strobolaryngoscopy showed mucosal hypertrophy in the front of bilateral laryngeal ventricles which covered the front of the vocal folds and anterior commissure during inspiration (**a**). It appeared excessive compensatory adduction of ventricular folds covering the glottis during phonation with normal morphology and movements of the vocal folds (**b**)

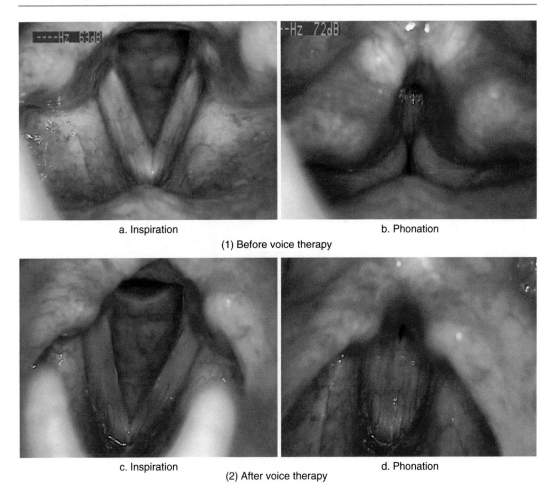

a. Inspiration   b. Phonation

(1) Before voice therapy

c. Inspiration   d. Phonation

(2) After voice therapy

Fig. 11.3 Functional dysphonia. (1) Before voice therapy: (**a**) Inspiration, (**b**) Phonation. (2) After voice therapy: (**c**) Inspiration, (**d**) Phonation. A 19-year-old male patient complained of aphonia during either attempted phonation or cough. Before voice therapy, strobolaryngoscopy showed the morphology and movements of the larynx were normal. During phonation, excessive compensatory compression of ventricular folds covered the glottis (1) (Video 11.1). After voice therapy, the patient's voice returned to normal. Strobolaryngoscopy showed that the supraglottic compression disappeared and the mucosal waves of the vocal folds were normal during phonation (2) (Video 11.2)

Laryngeal Stenosis 12

Laryngeal stenosis refers to stenosis or atresia of laryngeal cavity caused by various causes, sometimes in combination with tracheal stenosis. Causes include laryngeal trauma, iatrogenic injury (endotracheal intubation), chemical and physical injury, systemic disease (immune system disease), specific infection, laryngeal masses, congenital malformations, neurological or idiopathic factors (Figs. 12.1, 12.2, 12.3, 12.4, and 12.5).

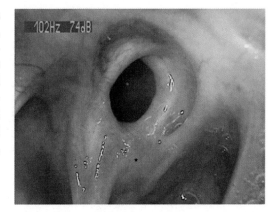

Fig. 12.1 Laryngopharyngeal stenosis. The shape of the epiglottis (*) was abnormal, and the laryngeal vestibule was annularly constricted. The scar formation involved the lingual surface of the epiglottis, lateral wall of pharynx, and posterior wall of pharynx

W. Xu, *Atlas of Strobolaryngoscopy*, https://doi.org/10.1007/978-981-13-6408-2_12

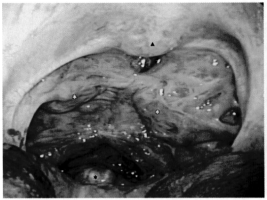

a. Oropharyngeal stenosis

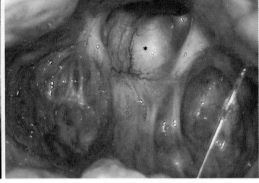

b. Laryngopharyngeal stenosis

Fig. 12.2 Laryngopharyngeal stenosis caused by caustic ingestion. (**a**) Oropharyngeal stenosis, (**b**) Laryngopharyngeal stenosis. Scarred stenosis involving the posterior wall of oropharynx and lateral wall of pharynx. Retropalatal

space disappeared. The scar formation presented at the tonsil (white *tonsils, ▲uvula, *epiglottis) (**a**). Scarred stenosis involved the hypopharynx with abnormal structure of the epiglottis (*) (**b**)

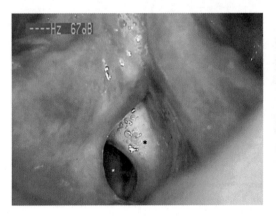

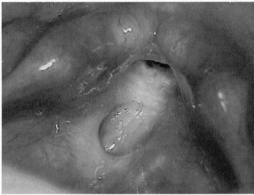

Fig. 12.3 Supraglottic stenosis caused by laryngeal tuberculosis. Strobolaryngoscopy showed cicatricial stenosis (*) involving in the supraglottic area, with normal morphology (white *) and limited movement of the vocal folds

Fig. 12.4 Laryngeal stenosis caused by previous surgical removal of recurrent laryngeal papilloma. A 14-year-old female patient complained of dyspnea and hoarseness after multiple surgical removal of laryngeal papilloma. Strobolaryngoscopy showed a glottic web involving the entire membranous portion of the vocal folds with scar formation in the glottis and supraglottis. The structure of the vocal folds was unclear

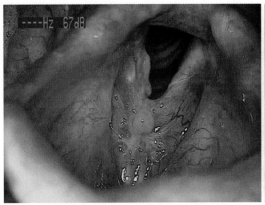

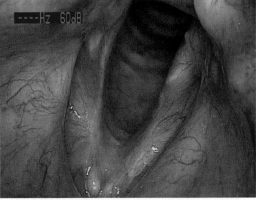

a. Preoperative view   b. Five months after microphonosurgery

Fig. 12.5 A glottic web caused by previous surgical removal of glottic carcinoma. (**a**) Preoperative view, (**b**) Five months after microphonosurgery. The patient had a glottic web caused by previous surgical removal of glottic carcinoma. Strobolaryngoscopy showed cicatricial adhesion at the anteromedian portion of bilateral vocal folds, irregular pseudomembrane and granulation hyperplasia locally, with absent mucosal waves during phonation (**a**). Five months after endoscopic web lysis and mucosal suturing of the vocal fold, the hoarseness relieved. Stroboslaryngoscopy showed improvement of glottic structure (**b**)

Vocal Fold Scar

13

Vocal fold scar is mainly due to weakened or disappeared vibration of the vocal folds caused by the disruption or obliteration of the distinctive layered structure of the vocal folds, which may be accompanied by glottal insufficiency, affecting the phonatory function. Congenital factors, trauma, infections, tumors, surgical injuries and other factors can lead to the formation of vocal fold scars, which should be avoided by surgeons during operations (Figs. 13.1 and 13.2; Video 13.1).

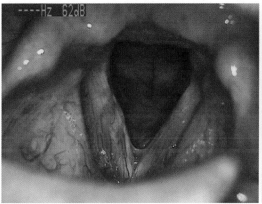
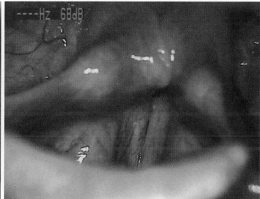

a. Inspiration

b. Phonation

Fig. 13.1 Vocal fold scar from previous right vocal fold polypectomy. (**a**) Inspiration, (**b**) Phonation. The patient had hoarseness which aggravated 2 months after right vocal fold polypectomy. Strobolaryngoscopy showed that the right vocal fold was stiff and scarred with severely reduced mucosal wave during phonation (Video 13.1)

Electronic Supplementary Material The online version of this chapter (https://doi.org/10.1007/978-981-13-6408-2_13) contains supplementary material, which is available to authorized users.

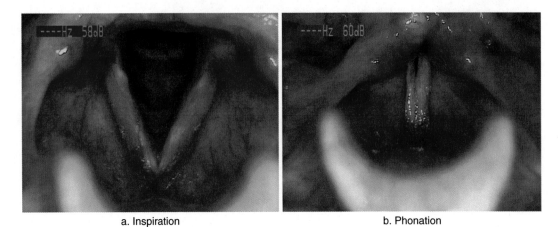

a. Inspiration   b. Phonation

Fig. 13.2 Bilateral vocal fold scar from previous phono-surgery for sulcus vocalis. (**a**) Inspiration, (**b**) Phonation. The patient had whispered for 18 months after surgery of bilateral vocal folds for sulcus vocalis. Strobolaryngoscopy showed that bilateral vocal folds were stiff with absent mucosal waves during phonation

Benign Tumors of the Larynx

14

The common benign tumors of the larynx are laryngeal papilloma, hemangioma, fibroma, lipoma and chondroma. The clinical symptoms vary in the size and location of the tumor. The early symptoms are atypical, including hoarseness, pharyngeal foreign body sensation or obstructive sensation. Hemoptysis can be presented in patients who have hemangioma. Dyspnea and/or dysphagia can be presented when laryngeal benign tumors get larger.

14.1 Laryngeal Papillomatosis

Laryngeal papillomatosis can occur in both children and adults and is induced by human papilloma virus (HPV). The juvenile laryngeal papillomatosis is the most common benign tumor of the larynx in children. The onset of juvenile form usually occurs at young age of less than 4 years old, and has much more diffuse extent, more aggressive, higher recurrence frequency than the adult form. They often lead to hoarseness and dyspnea, even life-threatening in severe cases. Adult-onset laryngeal papillomatosis has a malignant transformation tendency (Figs. 14.1, 14.2, 14.3, 14.4, and 14.5).

© Springer Nature Singapore Pte Ltd. and Peoples Medical Publishing House 2019
W. Xu, *Atlas of Strobolaryngoscopy*, https://doi.org/10.1007/978-981-13-6408-2_14

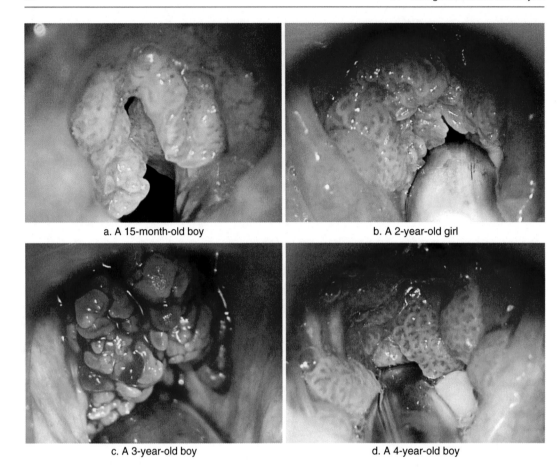

a. A 15-month-old boy   b. A 2-year-old girl

c. A 3-year-old boy   d. A 4-year-old boy

Fig. 14.1 Juvenile laryngeal papillomatosis (intraoperative view). (**a**) A 15-month-old boy, (**b**) A 2-year-old girl, (**c**) A 3-year-old boy, (**d**) A 4-year-old boy. All of the above children had different degrees of dyspnea and hoarseness. Laryngeal papillomatous mass which obstructed the airway was seen in intraoperative view

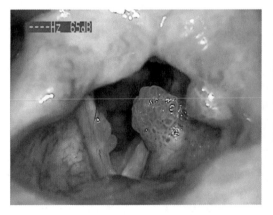

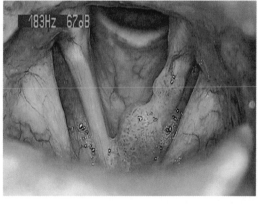

Fig. 14.2 Adult-onset laryngeal papillomatosis. Strobolaryngoscopy showed sporadic papillomas at the left ventricular fold, left arytenoid area and right vocal fold

Fig. 14.3 Adult-onset laryngeal papillomatosis. Strobolaryngoscopy showed papillomas at the left vocal fold

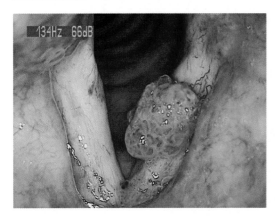

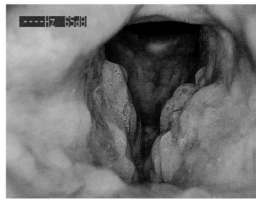

Fig. 14.4 Adult-onset laryngeal papillomatosis. Strobol-aryngoscopy showed papillomas at the left vocal fold

Fig. 14.5 Adult-onset laryngeal papillomatosis. Strobol-aryngoscopy showed diffuse bulging clusters of pink pap-illomas at the laryngeal surface of epiglottis, bilateral ventricular folds and bilateral vocal folds. Bilateral ven-tricular folds severely compressed during phonation with mucosal fluttering

14.2 Laryngopharyngeal Hemangioma

Laryngopharyngeal hemangiomas can occur at the soft palate, posterior or lateral pharyngeal wall, supraglottis, pyriform sinus. They occur mostly at the subglottis in the children. It can present with throat discomfort, pharyngeal foreign body sensation, hoarseness, hemoptysis, Purple-red mass can be seen at the involved region, which is easy to bleed (Figs. 14.6, 14.7, 14.8, and 14.9).

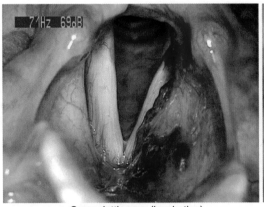

a. Supraglottic area (inspiration)

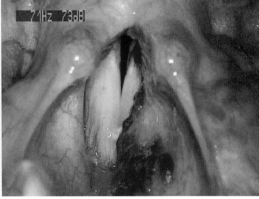

b. Supraglottic area (phonation)

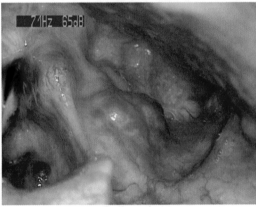

c. Pyriform sinus

Fig. 14.6 Laryngeal hemangioma involving the left side of supraglottic area. (**a**) Supraglottic area (inspiration), (**b**) Supraglottic area (phonation), (**c**) Pyriform sinus. A 40-year-old female patient had no specific discomfort. Strobolaryngoscopy showed a diffuse purple-red hemangioma at the left supraglottis, no abnormality at the glottis and the subglottis. The movements of bilateral vocal folds were normal

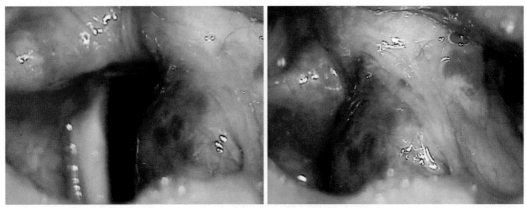

a. Before treatment

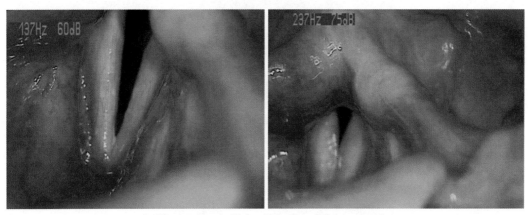

b. After treatment with local injection of pingyangmycin

Fig. 14.7 Laryngeal hemangioma involving the left side of supraglottic area. (**a**) Before treatment, (**b**) After treatment with local injection of pingyangmycin. A 41-year-old female patient had no specific discomfort. Strobolaryngoscopy showed a diffuse purple-red hemangioma at the left aryepiglottic fold which extended to the left arytenoid region and pyriform sinus, covering the left vocal fold. The movements of bilateral vocal folds were normal (**a**). After treatment with local injection of pingyangmycin, strobolaryngoscopy showed that the hemangioma at the supraglottic area had disappeared. Cicatricial change can be presented on the left ventricular fold (**b**)

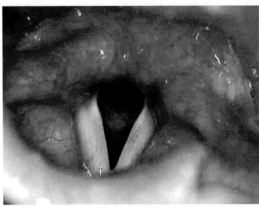

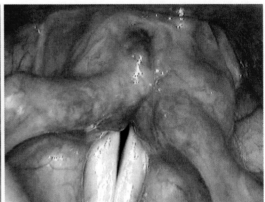

a. Inspiration

b. Phonation

Fig. 14.8 Hypopharyngeal hemangioma. (**a**) Inspiration, (**b**) Phonation. A 33-year-old female patient had pharyngeal foreign body sensation for 6 months.

Strobolaryngoscopy showed purple-red hemangioma at the interarytenoid region and posterior-lateral region of the left arytenoid

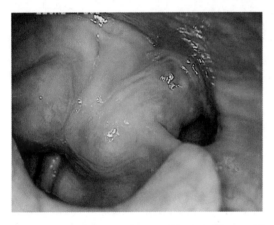

Fig. 14.9 Hypopharyngeal hemangioma. A 49-year-old female patient had pharyngeal foreign body sensation for 1 month. Strobolaryngoscopy showed purple-red hemangioma at the posterior-lateral region of the left arytenoid

14.3   Chondroma of the Larynx

Chondroma of the larynx is rare. Laryngeal chondroma and low-grade malignant laryngeal chondrosarcoma are the most common cartilaginous tumors. Laryngeal chondroma can occur in any cartilage of the larynx, mostly in the cricoid cartilage, followed by thyroid cartilage, arytenoid cartilage, and epiglottis. As most of laryngeal chondrosarcomas are low-grade malignant and have a slowly progressive growth pattern, laryngeal chondroma are often not easy to distinguish with laryngeal chondrosarcoma. Laryngeal chondroma is often less than 2–3 cm in diameter and can occur in both children and adults, while laryngeal chondrosarcoma is often larger than 3 cm in diameter and mostly occurs in the elderly aged 60–70 years old (Fig. 14.10).

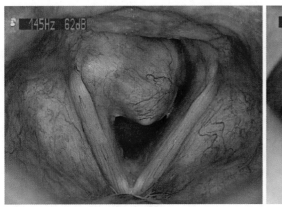
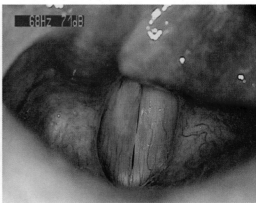

a. Inspiration   b. Phonation

Fig. 14.10 Laryngeal chondrosarcoma with dyspnea. (**a**) Inspiration, (**b**) Phonation. Female, 74 years old. Strobolaryngoscopy showed a smooth broad-base mass bulging under the right vocal process with normal vocal fold mobility. The patient had a laryngeal chondroma resection at the same area 12 years ago

Laryngeal Leukoplakia

15

Laryngeal leukoplakia mostly occurs at the vocal fold, also as known as the vocal fold leukoplakia. The vocal fold leukoplakia has a malignant transformation tendency and the histopathological features include squamous hyperplasia, mild dysplasia, moderate dysplasia, severe dysplasia, and carcinoma in situ. Its occurrence and development are related to the long-term effects of various pathogenic factors. The most common symptom of vocal fold leukoplakia is hoarseness, and mainly manifested as volatile or progressive hoarseness, throat discomfort, sore throat, and irritating cough (Figs. 15.1, 15.2, 15.3, 15.4, and 15.5).

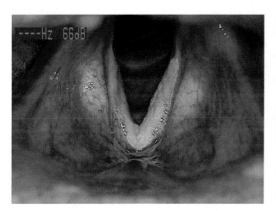

Fig. 15.1 Vocal fold leukoplakia with hyperkeratosis and hyperplasia. A 70-year-old male patient had intermittent hoarseness for 2 months. Strobolaryngoscopy showed that the entire left vocal fold, anterior commissure and the anterior portion of right vocal fold were covered with irregular white patches. The movements of bilateral vocal folds were normal but with moderately reduced mucosal wave during phonation

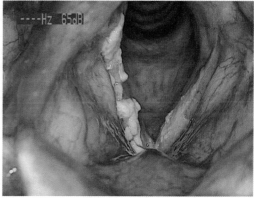

Fig. 15.2 Vocal fold leukoplakia with hyperkeratosis and parakeratosis. An 82-year-old male patient had persistent hoarseness for 4 months without a history of reflux. Strobolaryngoscopy showed that the entire right vocal fold, anterior commissure and the majority of left vocal fold were covered with white patches, worse on the right side with irregular protrusion. The mucosal wave of the right vocal fold was severely reduced and that of the left vocal fold was moderately reduced during phonation. The movements of bilateral vocal folds were normal

W. Xu, *Atlas of Strobolaryngoscopy*, https://doi.org/10.1007/978-981-13-6408-2_15

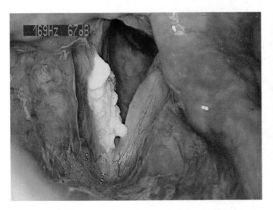

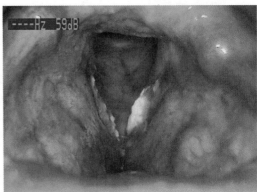

Fig. 15.3 Vocal fold leukoplakia with mild dysplasia. A 50-year-old male patient had persistent hoarseness for 5–6 years, aggravating for 2 months, and detection of vocal fold leukoplakia for 3 years. The patient had a history of chronic superficial gastritis for 15 years and had occasional acid reflux in the past 3 years. Strobolaryngoscopy showed a thick irregular white mass on the right vocal fold, with severely reduced mucosal wave but normal vocal fold mobility. No acid reflux was found by 24-h dual probe pH monitoring

Fig. 15.5 Laryngeal leukoplakia, severe dysplasia of the right vocal fold and carcinoma of the left vocal fold. A 44-year-old male patient had intermittent hoarseness for 3 months due to excessive smoking and alcohol intake. Strobolaryngoscopy showed irregular masses at the middle-posterior portion of bilateral vocal folds, with white patches on the surface. The lesion on the left side was more severe. The mucosal wave of the left vocal fold was absent and that of the right vocal fold was moderately reduced during phonation. The movements of bilateral vocal folds were normal

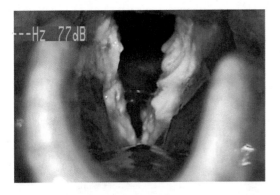

Fig. 15.4 Laryngeal leukoplakia with laryngopharyngeal reflux, mild to moderate dysplasia. A 57-year-old male patient had intermittent hoarseness for 1 year due to excessive smoking and alcohol intake, aggravating for 6 months. The patient had acid reflux occasionally. Strobolaryngoscopy showed thick irregular white protrusions involving bilateral vocal folds and the medial region of right arytenoid, with absent mucosal waves and normal vocal fold mobility. Esophageal 24-h pH monitoring detected 28 episodes of laryngopharyngeal reflux (8 episodes of acid reflux), 49 episodes of gastroesophageal reflux (45 episodes of acid reflux). The DeMeester score was 40.4

Malignant Tumors

16

Malignant tumors of the pharynx and larynx are mainly belonging to squamous cell carcinoma. The symptoms varied including hoarseness, dysphagia and dyspnea, depending on the involved location. Cervical lymph node metastasis and other signs involving the adjacent organs can also be presented. Symptoms tend to progressively aggravate in a short term.

16.1 Malignant Tumors of the Larynx

Laryngeal carcinoma is the most common among the malignant tumors of the larynx. Laryngeal carcinoma could be divided into three types based on the involved location: supraglottic carcinoma, glottis carcinoma and subglottic carcinoma. For supraglottic carcinoma and subglottic carcinoma, there are no obvious symptoms in the early stage while for the glottic carcinoma, hoarseness is often the first symptom in the early stage (Figs. 16.1, 16.2, 16.3, 16.4, 16.5, 16.6, 16.7, 16.8, and 16.9; Video 16.1).

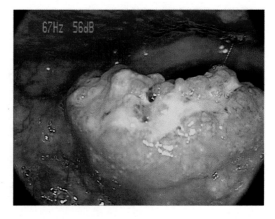

Fig. 16.1 Supraglottic carcinoma. The patient had odynophagia without hoarseness for 3 months. Strobolaryngoscopy showed rough and irregular mass at the epiglottis, with ulcers and necrosis on the surface

Electronic Supplementary Material The online version of this chapter (https://doi.org/10.1007/978-981-13-6408-2_16) contains supplementary material, which is available to authorized users.

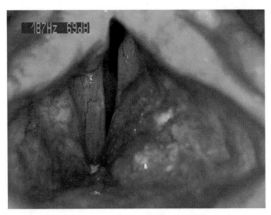

a. Observation under normal white light

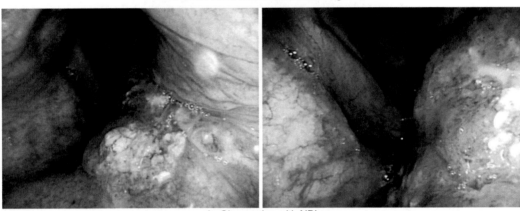

b. Observation with NBI

Fig. 16.2 Supraglottic carcinoma. (**a**) Observation under normal white light, (**b**) Observation with NBI. Observation under normal white light: endoscopy showed local roughness and irregular epithelial neoplasm involving the laryngeal surface of the epiglottis and the left ventricular fold (**a**). Observation with NBI: endoscopy presented abnormal mucosal microvasculature as tortuous and branch-like shapes in addition to scattered brown spots on the tumor surface (**b**)

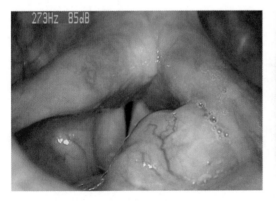

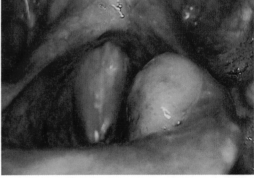

Fig. 16.3 Laryngeal adenoid cystic carcinoma. The patient had sore throat and persistent hoarseness for 1 year. Strobolaryngoscopy showed reddish nodular mass at the laryngeal surface of the epiglottis, left ventricular fold and left laryngeal ventricle. The morphology and movements of the bilateral vocal folds were normal

Fig. 16.4 Laryngeal carcinoid tumor. The patient had intermittent sore throat at the left side, which radiated to the ipsilateral ear for 4 years, aggravating for 6 months. Strobolaryngoscopy showed a reddish round mass at the left laryngeal surface of epiglottis. The morphology and movements of the bilateral vocal folds were normal

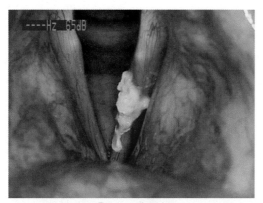

a. Preoperative view

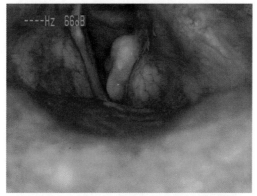

b. Forty days after CO_2 laser left cordectomy

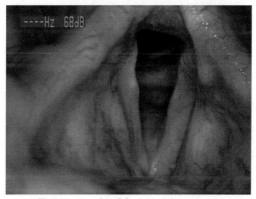

c. Three years after CO_2 laser left cordectomy

Fig. 16.5 Glottic carcinoma (left side). (**a**) Preoperative view, (**b**) Forty days after CO_2 laser left cordectomy, (**c**) Three years after CO_2 laser left cordectomy. A 72-year-old male patient had persistent hoarseness for 2 months. Before surgery, strobolaryngoscopy showed a broad-base irregular white neoplasm at the anterior-middle surface and edge of the left vocal fold. The mucosal wave of the left vocal fold was severely reduced during phonation. The vocal fold moved normally (**a**). Forty days after CO_2 laser left cordectomy, strobolaryngoscopy showed local granuloma formation at the left vocal fold (**b**). Three years after CO_2 laser left cordectomy, strobolaryngoscopy showed local scar formation and stiffness of the left side (**c**)

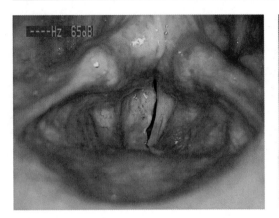

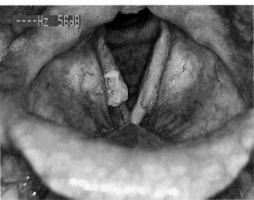

Fig. 16.6 Glottic carcinoma (right side). A 44-year-old male patient had persistent hoarseness for 4 months. Strobolaryngoscopy showed a rough neoplasm involving the right vocal fold, with severely reduced mucosal wave and normal vocal fold movement (Video 16.1)

Fig. 16.7 Glottic carcinoma (right side). The patient had hoarseness with no inducement for 6 months. Strobolaryngoscopy showed papillary neoplasm in the right vocal fold, with absent mucosal wave and normal vocal fold movement

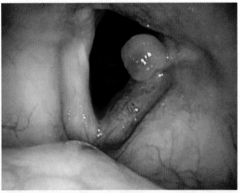

a. Observation under normal white light

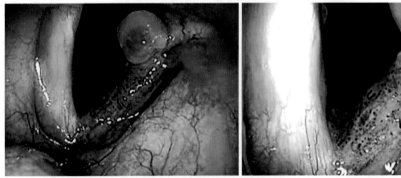

b. Observation with NBI

Fig. 16.8 Carcinoma and contact granuloma of the left vocal fold. (**a**) Observation under normal white light, (**b**) Observation with NBI. A 63-year-old female patient had intermittent hoarseness for 4 years after vocal overuse, aggravating to progressively persistent hoarseness for 3 months. Observation under normal white light: endoscopy showed the left vocal fold was congested and the mucosa was rough. A smooth granulomatous hyperplasia was seen at the left vocal process (**a**). Observation with NBI: endoscopy presented abnormal brown thick spots and branch-like angiogenesis on the surface and edge of left vocal fold and anterior commissure (**b**)

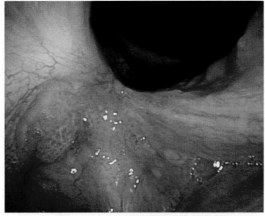

a. Observation under normal white light

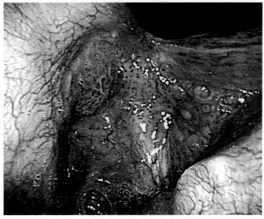

b. Observation with NBI

Fig. 16.9 Endoscopic view of laryngeal carcinoma. (**a**) Observation under normal white light, (**b**) Observation with NBI. Observation under normal white light: endoscopy showed the glottal web with the mucosal surface slightly thickening which was more obvious at the right side (**a**). Observation with NBI: endoscopy presented abnormal brown thick spots angiogenesis on the surface of the web, which was obvious at the right posterior part and anterior commissure (**b**)

16.2   Carcinoma of the Hypopharynx

The hypopharyngeal carcinoma is less common than laryngeal carcinoma, which mostly occurs at the pyriform sinus, followed by the posterior wall of the hypopharynx and the postcricoid region. Patients with the hypopharyngeal carcinoma do not present with many specific symptoms in the early stage. Some of them present with symptoms of pharyngeal foreign body sensation, swallowing discomfort and sore throat, which are prone to being misdiagnosed as chronic pharyngitis (Fig. 16.10).

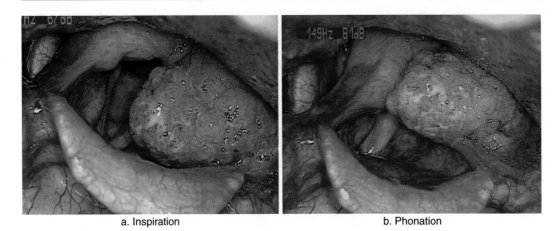

a. Inspiration   b. Phonation

Fig. 16.10 Carcinoma of the hypopharynx with immobility of the left vocal fold. (**a**) Inspiration, (**b**) Phonation. The patient had pharyngeal foreign body sensation at the left side for more than 1 month, accompanied by swallowing discomfort. Strobolaryngoscopy showed a cauliflower-like neoplasm at the left pyriform sinus with fixation of the left vocal fold at the paramedian position

Further Reading

1. Blitzer A, Brin MF, Stewart CF. Botulinum toxin management of spasmodic dysphonia (laryngeal dystonia): a 12-year experience in more than 900 patients. Laryngoscope. 1998;108:1435–41.
2. Cantarini L, Vitale A, Brizi MG, et al. Diagnosis and classification of relapsing polychondritis. J Autoimmun. 2014;48–49:53–9.
3. Cohen SM, Kim J, Roy N, et al. Prevalence and causes of dysphonia in a large treatment-seeking population. Laryngoscope. 2012;122:343–8.
4. Cohen SM, Pitman MJ, Noordzij JP, et al. Evaluation of dysphonic patients by general otolaryngologists. J Voice. 2012;26:772–8.
5. Cui W, Xu W, Yang Q, et al. Clinical features and surgical treatment for Chinese juvenile onset current respiratory papillomatosis (JORRP). Eur Arch Otorhinolaryngol. 2017;274:925–9.
6. Daya H, Hosni A, Bejar-Solar I, et al. Pediatric vocal fold paralysis: a long-term retrospective study. Arch Otolaryngol Head Neck Surg. 2000;126:21–5.
7. Dobbie AM, White DR. Laryngomalacia. Pediatr Clin North Am. 2013;60:893–902.
8. Ford CN, Inagi K, Khidr A, et al. Sulcus vocalis: a rational analytical approach to diagnosis and management. Ann Otol Rhinol Laryngol. 1996;105:189–200.
8. Franco RA, Singh B, Har-EI G. Laryngeal chondroma. J Voice. 2002;16:92–5.
10. Goudy S, Bauman N, Manaligod J, et al. Congenital laryngeal webs: surgical course and outcomes. Ann Otol Rhinol Laryngol. 2010;119:704–6.
11. Han DM, Sataloff RT, Xu W. Voice medicine. 2nd ed. Beijing: People's Medical Publishing House (China); 2017.
12. Hirano M. Morphological structure of the vocal cord as a vibrator and its variations. Folia Phoniatr. 1974;26:89–94.
13. Hoffman HT, Overholt E, Karnell M, et al. Vocal process granuloma. Head Neck. 2001;23:1061–74.
14. Hsiung MW, Woo P, Wang HW, et al. A clinical classification and histopathological study of sulcus vocalis. Eur Arch Otorhinolaryngol. 2000;257:466–8.
15. Hu R, Xu W, Liu H, et al. Laryngeal chondrosarcoma of the arytenoid cartilage presenting as bilateral vocal fold immobility: a case report and literature review. J Voice. 2014;28:129.e13–7.
16. Isenberg JS, Crozier DL, Dailey SH. Institutional and comprehensive review of laryngeal leukoplakia. Ann Otol Rhinol Laryngol. 2008;117:74–9.
17. Jacobson BH, Johnson A, Grywalski C, et al. The Voice Handicap Index (VHI): development and validation. Am J Speech Lang Pathol. 1997;6:66–70.
18. Lorenz RR. Adult laryngotracheal stenosis: etiology and surgical management. Curr Opin Otolaryngol Head Neck Surg. 2003;11:467–72.
19. Mat MC, Sevim A, Fresko I, et al. Behçet's disease as a systemic disease. Clin Dermatol. 2014;32:435–42.
20. Milczuk HA, Smith JD, Everts EC. Congenital laryngeal webs: surgical management and clinical embryology. Int J Pediatr Otorhinolaryngol. 2000;52:1–9.
21. Novakovic D, Waters HH, D'Elia JB, et al. Botulinum toxin treatment of adductor spasmodic dysphonia: longitudinal functional outcomes. Laryngoscope. 2011;121:606–12.
22. Peak W. Stroboscopy. San Diego: Plural Publishing; 2010. 3–7.
23. Pribitkin E, Friedman O, O'Hara B, et al. Amyloidosis of the upper aerodigestive tract. Laryngoscope. 2003;113:2095–101.
24. Prowse S, Knight L. Congenital cysts of the infant larynx. Int J Pediatr Otorhinolaryngol. 2012;76:708–11.
25. Rubin AD, Hawkshaw MJ, Moyer CA, et al. Arytenoid cartilage dislocation: a 20-year experience. J Voice. 2005;19:687–701.
26. Sama A, Carding PN, Price S, et al. The clinical features of functional dysphonia. Laryngoscope. 2001;111:458–63.
27. Sataloff RT. Autologous fat implantation for vocal fold scar. Curr Opin Otolaryngol Head Neck Surg. 2010;18:503–6.
28. Sataloff RT. Professional voice: the science and art of clinical care. 4th ed. San Diego: Plural Publishing; 2017.
29. Sataloff RT, Abaza M, Abaza NA, et al. Amyloidosis of the larynx. Ear Nose Throat J. 2001;80:369–70.
30. Schaefer SD. Management of acute blunt and penetrating external laryngeal trauma. Laryngoscope. 2014;124:233–44.

© Springer Nature Singapore Pte Ltd. and Peoples Medical Publishing House 2019
W. Xu, *Atlas of Strobolaryngoscopy*, https://doi.org/10.1007/978-981-13-6408-2

31. Spielmann PM, Palmer T, McClymont L. 15-Year review of laryngeal and oral dysplasias and progression to invasive carcinoma. Eur Arch Otorhinolaryngol. 2010;267:423–7.

32. Wang LM, Zhu Q, Ma T, et al. Value of ultrasonography in diagnosis of pediatric vocal fold paralysis. Int J Pediatr Otorhinolaryngol. 2011;75:1186–90.

33. Weller MD, Nankivell PC, McConkey C, et al. The risk and interval to malignancy of patients with laryngeal dysplasia; a systematic review of case series and meta-analysis. Clin Otolaryngol. 2010;35:364–72.

34. Woodbury K, Smith LJ. Relapsing polychondritis: a rare etiology of dysphonia and novel approach to treatment. Laryngoscope. 2011;121:1006–8.

35. Xu W, Han D, Hou L, et al. Value of laryngeal electromyography in diagnosis of vocal fold immobility. Ann Otol Rhinol Laryngol. 2007;116:576–81.

36. Xu W, Han D, Hu H, et al. Endoscopic mucosal suturing of vocal fold with placement of stent for the treatment of glottic stenoses. Head Neck. 2009;31:732–7.

37. Xu W, Han D, Hu R, et al. Characteristics of vocal fold immobility following endotracheal intubation. Ann Otol Rhinol Laryngol. 2012;121:689–94.

38. Xu W, Han D, Li H, et al. Application of the Mandarin Chinese version of the Voice Handicap Index. J Voice. 2010;24:702–7.

39. Xu W, Wang L, Zhang L, et al. Manifestation and treatment of lipoid proteinosis in larynx. Zhonghua Er Bi Yan Hou Tou Jing Wai Ke Za Zhi. 2010;45:301–4.

40. Xu W, Wang L, Zhang L, et al. Otolaryngological manifestations and genetic characteristics of lipoid proteinosis. Ann Otol Rhinol Laryngol. 2010;119:767–71.

41. Yang Q, Xu W, Li Y, et al. Value of laryngeal electromyography in spasmodic dysphonia diagnosis and therapy. Ann Otol Rhinol Laryngol. 2015;124:579–83.

42. Yiu EM, Lau VC, Ma EP, et al. Reliability of laryngo-stroboscopic evaluation on lesion size and glottal configuration: a revisit. Laryngoscope. 2014;124:1638–44.

43. Ylitalo R, Ramel S. Gastroesophagopharyngeal reflux in patients with contact granuloma: a prospective controlled study. Ann Otol Rhinol Laryngol. 2002;111:178–83.

Printed in the United States
By Bookmasters